Nursing  Cardio

A Collection of Reader-Submitted Medical Stories

Kerry Hamm

Disclaimer:

Names, locations, and portions of the
details included in this book have been altered
to protect the privacy of those involved.

<u>Warning:</u>

This edition features light profanity that may be offensive to some readers. The profanity has been used sparingly and in each instance the usage was included in the submission. I have chosen to leave some of these words in to emphasize portions of the stories.

By now, I am sure you are all too familiar with my *Real Stories from a Small-Town ER* series, which were collections of stories told to you from my time as a registration clerk in Ohio. If you are new here, don't fret! You don't have to worry about a 'certain order' for *any* of my books, including this one!

I have since moved on from the hospital scene, but that hasn't stopped readers from submitting stories of their own experiences from the medical field. Over time, I have received hundreds of stories-some funny, some sad, some downright scary or grotesque-and have worked with my readers to bring these stories to you in a follow up to my last *Real Stories* volume.

If I've learned anything from writing my series and compiling this book, it's that none of us are alone. We're all proof that we've seen some seriously messed up things out there, right? We have seen the good. We've seen the bad. We've seen the downright vile and disgusting. And then, we've seen the humor in these situations and we've been fortunate enough to share them with one another. There is a certain peace in knowing that as no matter how crazy we feel, we have formed solidarity amongst ourselves, knowing that for every bad day you've had, others have had them too. We have worked through the challenges of getting up and facing another drug seeker, another child abuse case, another young death, and another 'how the heck did that even happen?' moment together. You guys are not alone, and this book reaffirms that.

Several of the stories have been edited to bring you clear-cut and clean versions of tales submitted by loyal readers. I have done my very best to edit out hospital and town names, and in some cases my submitters wished to withhold their initials and other details from publication or requested that I edit stories for grammar/spelling. Some stories have been edited for length. I do my very best to preserve a reader's humor and emotions, as well as capture the reader's personality when I edit these submissions.

Though some of the stories in this collection are horrifying, I am glad none of us are alone in what we've witnessed or experienced.

Cheat Sheet

Some readers have been confused about terms used in this series. Here's a quick list to help you out!

LEO: Law Enforcement Officer

ETOH: shorthand for Ethyl Alcohol or Ethanol; commonly used to describe intoxicated individuals

Bus/Rig/Truck: Ambulance

M.D.: Medical Doctor

R.N.: Registered Nurse

MVA: Motor Vehicle Accident

EMS: Emergency Medical Services

EMT: Emergency Medical Technician

PD/FD: Police Department/Fire Department

D.A.: District Attorney

BOLO: Be on (the) Lookout

DCFS/CPS: Department of Children and Family Services/Child Protective Services

SNF: Skilled Nursing Facility. This can be a nursing home or one of many facilities for patients in need of supervised care

AMA: Against Medical Advice

LWBS/LBT: Left Without Being Seen/Left Before Triage

LOL: Little Old Lady

Breaking and ~~Entering~~...Uh, Just Breaking

I also work at a small-town ER and can verify to any disbelievers that the outrageous and unbelievable events that happen in your books do indeed happen in real life. This story is one of many that I could share with you.

At the time, I was on night shift, which is when things get weird. That night, we had seen a great number of jail clearances, ETOHs, ODs, and violent patients. We had also seen our frequent flyers, so, needless to say, we were quite tired. I'm going to play the victim here for a moment and tell you nobody was as exhausted as I was.

Let me tell you why.

My patient was an intoxicated, belligerent, abusive male in his late-twenties. We did not have the luxury of having our security guards present, so we had to steal two of our already-swamped orderlies to stand guard outside the patient's room. He spit on me, threatened my life, threatened my immediate safety, screeched like a banshee on fire, and was a thorn in my side like no other. His obnoxious behavior escalated quickly, and when he was denied a prescription for opioids, he then urinated on my scrub pants and new $200 clogs. It was at this point that we called the police.

The patient knew we notified law enforcement, so of course he did not wish to stick around. We could not legally restrain him—and quite frankly, we were fed up with his behavior—so none of us tried to stop him after he signed voluntary discharge papers. As far as we knew, the patient had left hospital property. Officers checked the front-entrance parking lot and confirmed that the man was hanging around.

Shortly after officers left the hospital, we were prepping for an incoming Code Blue. The patient en route was a child. Her mother checked on her during a late-night visit to the refrigerator, only to discover the toddler was not breathing—every parent's worst nightmare. It was an 'all hands on deck' scenario, one that took precedence over scratchy throats and finger pain.

As the ambulance was entering the bay, we heard a loud banging sound from our back entrance. We couldn't be bothered, so we tried to ignore the racket. Surely, if a hospital staff member had locked him or herself outside, they could walk their happy behinds around the building and enter through the public entryway.

The banging continued as we administered chest compressions to this lifeless child. We were on edge and the noise was causing further irritation and stress to staff and to the child's mother, who was standing in the corridor in obvious duress.

Our house supervisor pointed at me and said, "Go find out who that is out there, and tell them I want to see them in my office as soon as we save this child!"

I made my way to the metal emergency exit door, but as I neared, I could hear a male shouting. The closer I came to the door, I could recognize the voice. It was my unruly patient from earlier.

Because I could identify the man's voice, I did not want to open the door. Instead, I backed away. I saw a nurse sitting on the floor down a side hall just off the ER. She was sobbing and when I approached her, she told me that she left the Code Blue room to 'hide and cry,' because the child's death had been called and this pediatric nurse from upstairs did not want the child's mother to see her having a breakdown. I felt horrible, but I had no other option but to ask the nurse to keep an eye on the door. I instructed her to prevent staff from opening the door, and I informed her I was going to call law enforcement.

After I notified the police department, I wanted to inform our house supervisor, but she was in a consult room, speaking with the mother of our deceased child. I followed protocol by attempting to notify our security department by phone, but there was no answer. One of my coworkers stated she saw a security guard enter the office, so I thought I would go knock on the door, believing maybe the guard did not answer my call because he was on the line with another department.

I knocked on the door and was let in immediately. I notified the guard of the situation and he started typing at one of the keyboards until he pulled up security footage of the back portion of the emergency room.

There was my intoxicated patient, repeatedly hitting the emergency exit door with a wooden baseball bat. Despite the temperature being a mere 20-degrees, the man was not wearing a shirt or shoes. The footage did not have audio, but it was clear that the man was still screaming.

I was just about to leave the room and return to my post, when the tip of the ball bat bounced off the door and smacked the patient in the face.

One-two-three-knockout!

This man was down for the count, and how couldn't he be? Not only did he hit himself in the face with a baseball bat, but he also appeared to have hit his head on the dumpster as he went down. He didn't fall gracefully, either, so it wasn't like what you see in the movies; this patient did not slowly, gently, or dramatically fall to the concrete. This man hit himself in the face, hit the back of his head on the dumpster, and then hit the side of his head on the concrete in a matter of seconds. Really, it was just *boom, boom, boom.*

You may think I am a witch for this, but my first instinct was to laugh. I mean, if you recall, I had to change out of my scrub pants and disinfect my new shoes. So yeah, as I was standing in my Mickey Mouse scrub top with mismatched Winnie the Pooh scrub bottoms, I did laugh at this man receiving the karma he so desperately deserved.

As hateful as I am for laughing, I am still a dedicated nurse. Even as a child, my passion was caring for others. I could not leave this man unconscious in the middle of the night, and especially in cold weather.

I hurried out of the security office and managed to find three nurses and techs to help me out. We were going to lift the patient to a gurney and wheel him to a room. Police officers would be there any second, and we were confident that officers would restrain the patient during treatment.

None of us remembered that the emergency exit was equipped with an alarm, so when we opened it, a loud ringing filled the ER. Alarms in switchboard and security went off as well, which prompted the switchboard operator to notify the fire department. Realizing our blunder, we attempted to move the gurney and close the door, but the gurney was stuck in the doorframe.

It was just my luck that I was trapped outside with the man, who was bleeding from a head wound. To make matters worse, I suffer from extreme nervousness, so when I realized the man could come to at any moment—and because I knew he was violent—my nerves kicked into overdrive and I felt the need to urinate.

I was pushing the gurney while my coworkers were pulling, when I heard a noise behind me. Thinking it was the patient regaining consciousness, I screamed and peed my pants. I am absolutely humiliated to let you know it was just a cat trying to jump into the dumpster.

We eventually moved the gurney inside and transported the patient to our ER by the old-fashioned backboard method.

This patient cracked the bridge of his nose and required a bandage to the superficial gash to the back of his head, but otherwise was in decent physical condition. He was too dazed from the incident to react violently when he came to, thank goodness.

Officers identified the patient as a wanted fugitive, so he was arrested and transported to jail as soon as we wrapped up his treatment.

--A.M.
Michigan

Time of the Season

Sometimes, ER workers will never know the 'whole story.' Here's an example:

I am 72. Last Fall, I thought I was having a mini-stroke. I had some symptoms that were just enough to make me nervous, but they were not severe.

When my tongue started to get a bit numb, I decided to go to the ER. I chose to go by myself, just because my son would have probably just freaked out at the hospital.

At the hospital, the examining doctor told me I did not fit the profile for a mini-stroke, but still suggested blood tests. Instead of shelling out tons of money on an uncertainty—and for symptoms I could live with, at least for the moment—I declined and decided to just go home and sleep off whatever it was. If my symptoms worsened, I could always come back. If they went away, I could rest easy, knowing I wouldn't have a bill.

The next morning, my teenage grandson greeted me and asked if I had enjoyed the 'special' cupcake he had given me the night before.

I was shocked when I had put two and two together! I mean, what?!

My grandson and I have a special bond. We have discussed how I am a child of the sixties and how grandma used to enjoy 'special' brownies.

Well, my grandson decided to help me relive some of my days-gone-by. He thought he was making me happy.

We had a very serious discussion about the fact that, while I have no moral objections to 'special' edibles, there are some things that are still a big no-no.

I told him, "Next time, let me know, so I can at least enjoy it!"

I am so glad I declined those blood tests!

--R.K.P.

<u>Another Brick in the Wall</u>

It was my first day on the job as a Basic, and throughout the day, I found myself questioning my career choice. I doubted my ability to do anything right, especially after I found myself doing everything wrong. My partner, a seasoned medic, seemed irritated with me, and my anxiety was through the roof. At one point, when we stopped at a gas station for lunch, I thought about calling for an Uber and leaving him to do the job himself. I figured it'd be better for him to work alone than to work with some girl who had no idea what she was doing.

Well, I didn't have time to ditch my partner because we were contacted by dispatch to respond to a complaint of 'trapped in building.' It was a 5F commercial (five flights of stairs in a commercial, non-residential building), so that had my skin crawling, too. I'd transported patients down stairs in training, but never in a real situation. I was sure I was going to drop this patient, if we had to move him down the stairs.

Honestly, the whole ride there, I thought the call was something the fire department should have responded to, not EMS. As soon as we arrived and found our patient, though, it was crystal clear as to why we were called.

Inside this abandoned building, on the second floor, a man was standing with his face to the brick wall. His pants were down around his ankles. All I could focus on was his bare ass. As much as I didn't want to look, I couldn't help it. The moon was out, and boy, was it full!

Admittedly, I was feeling scared when we came upon the man. I mean, we were in a condemned building. It was bright outside, but the room we were in was rather dark because there were only a few windows that weren't boarded up. The man's hands were not visible, and he did not immediately speak to us or turn to acknowledge our presence.

My partner was a no-nonsense kind of guy, so he got right to it and asked, "You the guy who called 911?"

The man at the wall nodded but didn't speak.

"It's not cool to call 911 just to waste our time," my partner said with a grunt. "If you called us in here to rob us, you're not going to get much."

"I'm not gonna hurt anyone," the man sniffled. "I need help, man. I really messed up. I need help."

"Are you holding a weapon?" I blurted out.

The man sobbed and said, "Oh, man! You brought a chick?"

"Are you holding a weapon or not?" my partner demanded.

"I ain't got a weapon," the man cried. "I told y'all, I just need help."

My partner asked the man to slowly lift his hands, just so we could feel safer about moving closer. The man lifted his hands above his head and was only holding a cell phone.

When we moved to the sides of this man, we realized he really was trapped *in* the building. His penis was stuck in a hole in the wall.

I had no idea how to react, but my partner—who'd not cracked a smile all shift—started laughing his ass off.

"Oh, come on, man," the patient nagged. "It ain't funny. I need help."

We gloved up and tried to remove the patient's penis from the wall, but he was…ahem…balls deep in the hole. We did our best to treat his appendage with the greatest care, but he cried out in pain a few times. Not only was he stuck, but as we tried to pull and wiggle his 'not-so-little man,' the bricks surrounding his penis rubbed his skin and he sustained scrapes and papercut-like lacerations.

It took 30 minutes to free the man from the wall. The metal piercing that he had in the tip of his penis had caught on something inside the wall, which left him stuck.

Against better judgment, I asked the man why he would stick his penis in the wall in the first place. He said he had a 'condition' and he thought the wall was 'sexy.'

Umm…Yeah, I didn't know how to respond to that. (I looked it up later and apparently some people are attracted to inanimate objects.)

The patient refused treatment or medical transport. He asked us not to tell anyone what happened, but of course, I'm telling you and still tell all the new Basics about that day.

My partner asked if I wanted to go out for drinks after our shift ended, and he was a lot nicer then. He gave me advice for the job and encouraged me to continue in the career, and I did.

Next month will be my 10th anniversary with our station.

--M.L.
Indiana

Bad Timing

This wasn't a shining star moment in my career, but it happened and there's nothing I can do to change it.

We received a patient following an MVA. The patient had been severely intoxicated while riding an ATV, when he lost control of the vehicle and flipped it. The ATV went airborne before it landed on the patient. He presented to us in critical condition. I know it's sad to say, but we all knew there was simply no way he could survive his injuries. Still, we tried to save him.

The patient passed away after a few minutes in our ED. We tried, God knows we did, but there was nothing we could do. It was simply out of our hands.

Family came in the room to say their goodbyes to the patient, just as I was wrapping up. As a creature of habit, I pumped hand sanitizer from a bottle on the counter. I don't know what happened, really, but somehow, I managed to get hand sanitizer in my eye. Instinctively, I rubbed my eyes, forgetting I had sanitizer on my hands. I effectively blinded myself. My eyes were watering so much that it felt like I had Niagara Falls rushing down my cheeks.

I tried to leave the room as quickly as possible, since family members were crying in their moment of grief.

Well, when you're suddenly blinded, carrying out simple tasks are not as easy as they usually are.

First, I walked into the counter and stabbed myself in the stomach with the corner of the counter. The patient's family, from what I could gather, didn't notice much.

The family—and the entire ED—*did* notice when I tried running out of the room, only to run smack-dab into the glass door. As if that wasn't bad enough, I hit the door with such force that it came off its track and crashed to the floor. The sound of the door breaking was loud, and there was glass everywhere.

Some of the RNs in our working station were laughing. Some rushed to help. One of the patient's family members started laughing and couldn't stop, so this made his other family upset and they demanded he leave the room. In turn, he became angry at me and was shouting at me—while I basically stood still, afraid to move, and was still trying to get the sanitizer out of my eyes.

Luckily, I didn't get in any trouble. My supervisor said it was a poorly-timed accident.

I still feel horrible for interrupting the family's grieving.

--A.E.
Rhode Island

<u>The Calling</u>

We had this LOL (Little Old Lady) in a room down the hall, and she was the sweetest patient I think I'd ever met.

Well, after helping her put on her gown, I assisted her in bed and told her a doctor would be right with her. She was so polite and told me to tell the doctor to take his time, even though I know she was in pain.

A few minutes later, as I was charting, her call chime had gone off. I used the intercom to say, "Jane, do you need some help?"

She replied, "Well, yes! All these years I've been praying, and I'm so happy you've finally answered!"

I said, "Jane, what seems to be the problem?"

She started babbling about finances, her cat's declining health, and she wanted me to help her granddaughter succeed in culinary school. She was so sweet that I felt bad interrupting her.

"Jane," I asked, "who do you think you're speaking to right now?"

I could see her on the video footage from the camera in her room. She looked confused.

"Well, God, right?" she responded.

I couldn't help but to laugh.

"Jane," I said, "this is your nurse. You've hit the call button."

"The call-what?" she asked.

I went to Jane's room, and it turned out that she'd been on top her call button/remote control pad. She had accidentally called me when she rolled over.

Jane laughed it off and said, "Well, that explains a lot. You sounded awfully young to be God."

--C.T.
Georgia

<u>Priorities</u>

My partner and I were dispatched to a residence for a complaint of pregnancy complications and possible preterm labor.

Upon arriving, we met our patient, a woman in her late-30s. She could hardly speak to us because she was experiencing contractions roughly every one to four minutes. Her pre-teen daughter did most of the explaining and stated the patient had gone to the bathroom and noticed a concerning amount of blood. The patient took a breather and informed us that she felt a bulge extending from her vagina when she wiped.

Our patient was deeply concerned about her unborn child but was also concerned about her pre-teen. I informed the patient that her daughter could ride along with us. Per the patient's request, I then explained the procedure for transporting her and what I expected to happen once we arrived at the hospital.

I asked the patient to lie down on our stretcher, and she did.

"Let's get you loaded," I said.

I turned and looked for my partner. I didn't see him in any of the surrounding rooms. I called his name, but nope, nothing.

"Did you see the guy who came in with me?" I asked the patient and her daughter.

The daughter nodded and said, "Yeah, he had his phone out. Then he went outside."

I groaned because I knew what he was doing. He'd been playing that Pokémon game all day. It was like he was obsessed with it.

I walked outside and called my partner's name. No reply.

I walked to the end of the driveway and looked both ways down the street.

There was my partner, approximately a block and a half from the patient's home, standing in the middle of the street with his phone in his hand.

"Hey!" I shouted.

"One sec," he hollered back.

"No," I yelled. "You need to come now."

"Will you just give me a second?" he asked, clearly agitated.

"We need to go," I ordered. "Come on. Put your phone away and stop playing that stupid game."

My partner let out a loud roar and screamed, "You made me lose it!"

He complained the whole time he was walking back, the whole time we transported the patient, and the whole time back to the station.

Our patient's complaint was legitimate. That bulge she felt when she wiped was her water sac, and she was in preterm labor. Luckily, her newborn survived and was released after a few weeks on NICU.

I reported my partner's actions to my supervisor, and my partner was terminated immediately. I had not been the only employee to complain, and my supervisor said patients had also called to complain about my partner's behavior during runs in which I was not involved.

I honestly still can't believe that he chose a cell phone video game over patients requiring medical attention. Did he think he wouldn't be punished for his behavior, or did he just think the game was more important?

--Initials and location withheld at request

When my nurse saw me covered in mud, with a broken ankle, she asked, "You were part of the rodeo in town this weekend, huh?"

I lied. I flat-out lied. Sure was, rode a bull and everything.

Look, I was chasing a baby bunny, slipped when I ran through a puddle, and when I tried to get up, I slipped again.

I thought if I could catch the bunny, I could keep it as a pet. It got away, and I got a cast, some pain meds, and a hefty bill.

--O.Y.
Virginia

The first thing out of my doctor's mouth when he saw me was, "Late night BMX stunts?"

I said yes, but what really happened was I was trying to put on my pajama pants by jumping into both legs at the same time, tripped, and broke my arm when I fell.

I put on my boyfriend's (who was drunk and passed out just a few feet from where I fell) racing shirt because my shirt was too tight and was impossible to get on, and I drove myself to the ER.

--N.K.
Washington

Author's Note: Are you two sure you aren't related?

<u>I Need That!</u>

I work at a government hospital, on the inpatient substance rehab floor. Upon a patient's admission, we examine his/her personal belongings. Some people don't understand why we do this, but you'd be surprised by how sneaky people can be when they're entering rehab, especially if the admission was not of their own choice. For example, one patient purchased one of those hollowed-out tubes of toothpaste online and filled the bottom half of the tube with pills. I guess he thought we'd never notice. Other patients bring bottles of mouthwash, when we only allow mouthwash that is alcohol-free. This list goes on and on.

Well, one day I asked an incoming patient to place her luggage on the table for inspection. For several minutes, she refused. This, of course, is a red flag. Patients will use every excuse in the world to get out of inspection. They'll dig up a few more excuses if we find contraband items.

Anyway, I finally told the patient that she could either place her bag on the table for inspection, or she could be denied admission to our floor. I know it's harsh to threaten someone like that, especially because she'd served her country and had fallen on hard times, but I have an obligation to these patients to offer them the best healthcare—and that requires effort on their part. In this case, the patient could follow the rules or leave.

Finally, the patient slammed her bag on the table and started hovering over me as I went through her belongings—another red flag.

At one point, as I reached the bottom of the bag, the patient tried to snatch the luggage away from me. She said, "Okay, you've looked enough."

Here I was, thinking I was going to find a stash of drugs, but as I continued inspecting her belongings, I was surprised to see a first in my career.

The patient's luggage was lined with sex toys and condoms.

When I say sex toys, I don't mean she brought along a little pink vibrator.

This patient had life-like dildos with suction cups to hold them in place on a hard surface, fuzzy handcuffs, and even things I am too embarrassed to describe.

"Why did you bring this stuff?" I asked.

As far as I knew, the patient's file did not reference a sexual addiction, but I suspected she had an undiagnosed addiction when I saw all these things.

She looked at me like I was stupid when she explained that sex helped take her mind off drugs, so she thought she could have 'lots of it' (sex) with other patients while they were all battling addiction.

Phew.

I confiscated all the sex toys, condoms, and lubricants from the patient's luggage and explained our floor's strict policies regarding sexual conduct between patients.

The woman turned out to be a nightmare of a patient and voluntarily signed herself out. I never saw her again, but I hope she found the help she needed.

Since then, I've never found sex toys in anyone's luggage, so hopefully she was the only one to ever try to pull that off.

--I.P.

Texas

<u>Disgusting!</u>

I had registered a man for a complaint of constipation caused by medication that his PCP had prescribed.

Other than telling me that he had been backed up, the man seemed in good health and didn't appear to be in pain. Unfortunately for him, since he came to the emergency room on a day when we were seeing patients for chest pains, MVAs, and severe injuries stemming from assaults, he was sent to the waiting room and it looked like he'd have to be there for at least two hours, if not more.

The man came to my counter a few times and demanded to be seen. I explained to him everything I just told you. He was angry, but each time, he went back to the waiting room.

I'd say it was about two hours in that I saw the man go to the restroom. I didn't give it much more thought because, whatever, there's no law stopping someone from trying to poop.

Well, I was registering a stabbing victim, when I heard a woman scream from the waiting room. It was a blood-curdling scream like you hear in movies. Before that day, I've never heard anyone scream like that in real life.

Security was divided between the ICU and the back part of the ER, and my coworkers had gone to lunch. I was afraid that maybe someone keeled over in the waiting room, so I placed the stabbing victim on a bench and hit a call light that signaled 'immediate care needed,' and I walked toward the waiting room.

There were about 10-15 people, mostly women and children, fleeing the waiting room. It gave me chills because, usually, if a crowd is moving away from something, it's for good reason.

I peeked in there and saw the constipation patient drawing on the walls…using a piece of excrement that was so large that he couldn't fit his entire hand around.

"What the hell are you doing?" I shouted at him. "Is that poop? Are you drawing on the walls with poop?"

He shrugged and said, "You've kept me waiting for two hours, so how else am I supposed to keep busy? You call this an emergency room? People come to the emergency room to get in and out in fifteen minutes. You don't make someone sit for two hours."

I know I violated HIPAA, and I ordinarily wouldn't, but I yelled, "You checked in because you couldn't poop! The emergency room is for all the people who've been shot and stabbed today, not because you can't take a dump!"

I informed the man that I was calling the police, and I started walking away.

As soon as I got behind my counter and started dialing 911, the man came up and tossed his poop to me like he was throwing me a set of car keys.

This is the worst part.

Out of habit of people throwing pens and stuff to me, I caught his poop.

When the 911 operator answered, I was screaming and gagging. I don't know what she thought was going on, but she kept asking me questions and telling me to calm down.

My coworkers came back up front and saw me trying to get the poop off my hands and into a biohazard bag, since I couldn't throw it in our paper-only trash bin. It was really hard, because the biohazard bags are kept on a roll, and I was trying to hold the phone between my ear and shoulder, and then pull a bag down by using whichever fingertips that weren't contaminated.

I made my coworker take the call and report the patient, but he'd already left. Officers said they'd go talk to him, but I don't think they did. I don't know for sure.

Housekeeping was pissed to have to scrub poop off the walls, and I had to wash my hands about 1900 times before my shift ended.

I've never experienced anything like that, and I pray I never do again.

--R.K.
New Jersey

<u>Karma</u>

A few years back, we had this frequent who'd come in and always require a security escort off the property. He was obnoxious, rude, and always seemed to be looking for trouble. This patient had a detailed history of assaulting staff members (physically and verbally), and none of us wanted to be assigned as his nurse. We did not dislike *caring* for the patient, but we did dislike the conditions in which he forced us to care for him.

Most of the time, this patient's complaints were superficial, while often they were nonexistent and largely exaggerated. For example, this man once registered because he felt he could not remove the Band-Aid we had placed over a papercut he'd received. Yes, he indeed came back one day after receiving the Band-Aid, now demanding that we remove it. When we did, he called out in pain and started his typical threats of suing the facility for malpractice and unjust pain and suffering, all because we failed to shave the top of his hand before applying the Band-Aid over the papercut.

Yep, this guy was a real piece of work.

Well, the patient's obnoxious behavior escalated.

One time, I was in the room, checking his saline drip, when he blew an air horn. Apparently, you can buy pocket-sized canisters and carry them on your person. The patient said he was 'punishing' me because another nurse had failed to bring him an extra pillow in the time in which he believed he deserved it. (Pardon us for dealing with a seizing patient, right?) Boy, he scared the ever-living daylights out of me. I wanted to smack him, but I couldn't.

Well, the patient came in on a busy weekday and demanded to be seen ahead of patients presenting with broken limbs, severe abdominal pain/tenderness, and even asthmatic children. He said he felt like he might have diarrhea later, because he'd eaten a greasy lunch. I don't know what he wanted us to do about this, but when we expressed that his complaint was non-emergent, he claimed he had chest pains. By hospital protocol, we are required to take chest pains straight back, even if we know they're lying.

I drew straws and lost. It was my turn to be this patient's nurse. Yay, me.

When I entered the patient's room, he was being a butt. That was nothing unusual. A CNA was already in the room, setting up the EKG machine.

Test results showed what we already knew: the patient was fine.

I went back to the patient's room and said, "Well, it looks like your heart is in fine shape."

He responded, "I know. I'm here because I ate three cheeseburgers and I know I'm going to have the shits later."

I sighed and finally broke down. I explained that we were quite busy providing care to patients with *real* problems. The patient said he didn't care, that his Medicaid paid my salary, and that I needed to stop what I was doing and show him the attention he deserved.

I told the patient I did not have time for his antics today, but I would surely send in a doctor…when one became available.

As I was turning to leave, the patient demanded that I bring him an extra blanket.

I thought to myself that I would grab the blanket, just so we didn't have another episode of him standing in the corridor, screaming about how I'd forgotten to bring the blanket like he did a few weeks back, and then I would see if we could get a doctor to go in and get him out of our hair.

When I returned to the room with a blanket, the patient yelled at me because I did not bring him a glass of ice water.

"You didn't ask for ice water, John," I said. "You asked for a blanket. By the way, I'm a nurse, not a five-star hotel employee."

The patient became angry, and I thought he was going to assault me, by the way he jumped up out of his bed and reached in the pocket of his jeans.

I screamed, but before anyone could come to the room to help me, the patient was in my face. He extended his hand and blew. It all happened rather quickly. I clenched my eyes shut.

The patient started gagging and clutched my wrist. He was coughing, and I could tell it wasn't a staged cough for attention.

When I opened my eyes, my scrubs were covered in bright blue glitter. The patient was still coughing, and now he was doubled over.

Finally, the man hacked so much that he choked himself and vomited right down the front of his jeans and all over his shoes.

"I accidentally sucked in some of that glitter," he gasped, as two other nurses ran in the room to help.

According to the patient, he thought it would be funny to 'cover' me in glitter to 'ruin my day.'

After his plan backfired, he never caused us problems again. Actually, I think we only saw him twice after that, and both visits were something we in the healthcare field would deem 'acceptable' to come to the ER for, so it seemed he really straightened up and learned his lesson.

I know it's probably not the funniest thing I could share with you, but it was kind of the strangest thing I've encountered, and I really think it's fun to tell the story of the patient who got a taste of his own medicine.

--K.N.
Kentucky

<u>Carried Away</u>

I'm an RN on Oncology, so I was not home during the accident, but I was at the hospital when my father was brought to the ER via ambulance at 02:00. I was scared out of my mind when they told me my dad was experiencing altered mental status and that he had to be restrained due to trying to 'fight off' ER staff.

Immediately, I left my station and went down to the ER, where my father was tied to the bed with canvas straps. They'd started a drip to soothe him, and two doctors were ordering the unit clerk to page X-Ray and CAT Scan.

My father was a mess. His face was bloody, and it was clear his leg was broken.

Nobody would let me in the room at first, so I tried to call John, my 15-year-old son. I figured I had a better chance of reaching him, since it was a weekend and he stayed up until three in the morning playing video games, while my husband was asleep and wouldn't wake up even if a train crashed through the bedroom. A medic recognized me from family pictures at my home, and he informed me that my son would be riding to the hospital with my husband. What a mess. I never even thought that we'd have an accident like this at my house. We moved my dad in with us because we were terrified that something like this would happen at *his* house.

Finally, a nurse told me I could enter my father's room. She said he was still 'acting pretty weird,' and she said he was talking nonsense about dragons and flying.

I went in and sat by the bed. I took my father's hand and asked, "How are you feeling, Dad? Have the meds kicked in yet?"

He turned his head, and with a look of urgency in his eyes, he replied, "I have to get out of here. I need to talk to John."

"John's on the way," I told him.

He tried to sit up but couldn't.

"Stay still, Dad," I said, with tears in my eyes. "Everything's going to be okay."

"Tell John I found the dragon," he said. "I found the dragon."

"Dad, John's on his way. Let's just try to stay calm, okay?"

My father was insistent upon speaking to my son. At one point, he demanded that I call John and tell him not to come to the hospital. My dad went on and on about how he had been flying and found a dragon, about how the dragon wasn't in its lair, and then he started panicking over how much time was passing. Because he was getting riled up, my father's nurse came by and told me I needed to leave the room. I felt absolutely helpless.

Because of his babbling, there was an order for CAT Scan to check for any visible abnormalities. They wanted to do that before my father had his leg set.

My husband and son arrived. My husband asked how everything happened and asked if my dad was okay, but then he said he was going to the waiting room to sleep. My son was worried and said that he didn't know what had happened, that he only heard my father yell from upstairs, and then he heard a big crash. He found my father unconscious at the bottom of the stairs, and he called 911. He tried waking my husband, but he couldn't (go figure).

It wasn't until a good 20 minutes later that I was in the waiting room, talking to a nurse. She said my father was fighting his drip and was still waking up in a panicked state to talk about dragons. My son overheard and became excited.

"He found it?" he exclaimed.

I was so confused. "You know what he's talking about?"

John nodded. "Grandpa saw me playing my game, so he wanted to play. He's been helping me look. It's a super rare dragon that drops a mount."

My son may have well been speaking a foreign language to me, because all I took from that was it was part of some online computer game. I knew my dad had been spending lots of extra time on the computer in the spare bedroom, but he's always had a thing for online poker rooms, so I just assumed that's what he'd been up to.

When we got down to it, after my father was patched up and ready to be discharged, we learned he tried running downstairs to tell John about the rare dragon he found, when he tripped.

I couldn't believe it, but my father was more concerned with us getting John home (in hopes that the dragon would still be at that location) than he was about his own health.

John did not find the dragon that night. We did some switching around and gave my son the extra bedroom, just so we could give my father a room on the first floor.

My dad passed away last year, but he played that video game right up until he passed. I think it made him feel closer to John and also gave him a sense of purpose.

--A.E.
Virginia

An Innocent Emergency

We once responded to a 911 call from a young child. She wouldn't tell dispatch anything besides, "It's real bad, and they need help."

The call ended abruptly with an adult screaming, "Hey!" and dialing-back to the number from which the child called yielded no answer. My partner and I were dispatched to the residence listed for the landline, and we were to dispatch EMS, if necessary.

When we arrived at the residence, we noted a child, approximately 4 years of age, with a woman who appeared to be the child's mother. Mom was holding an infant, watching another infant play on a blanket spread on the front yard, and the little girl was drawing on the sidewalk with chalk. The little girl appeared overjoyed to see us. The child's mother appeared anything *but* overjoyed.

"Ma'am," I asked, as I approached the lawn, "is everything okay here today?"

She seemed confused and slowly answered, "Yes. Why?"

"Well," I said, "we received a 911 call from your residence."

"Jane!" the mother yelled at the little girl. "Did you call 911?"

The little girl nodded.

"Why did you call 911?" I asked the child. "Was someone hurt or in trouble?"

The child nodded again.

"Officer," the mother said, "I can assure you nobody at my house is or was hurt or in trouble. I'm home alone with my kids."

My partner asked the child why she called 911.

She pointed to the middle of the road and said, "The ice cream truck was broken. My mom said we couldn't get ice cream. Then, this big truck came and took the ice cream truck away."

"Oh my gosh," the mother groaned. "You called 911 when I told you to take the money back inside?"

"But it was *broken*," the little girl said. "And you said that if something bad happens, I should call for help."

"Well, I didn't mean to call 911 for *that*. You only call them if mommy hits her head or something."

The child's mother apologized profusely. She was embarrassed, but we told her not to worry about it. We were just glad that the family was safe.

I'm sure the mother had a long talk with her child about when to call 911.

--M.W.
Nevada

Talk about Embarrassing

My first year as an RN was horrible. While it's true that nurses and doctors eventually become like family to each other, I've noticed that new nurses aren't generally included in this family. In fact, I was treated so poorly by fellow nurses and staff that I would cry in the bathroom (when I'd actually be able to go to the bathroom), and most of my time away from work was spent dreading going back.

The social ostracism was difficult enough. Then, I was new to working in the emergency room setting. I started off on another wing, one that didn't require nearly as much movement and urgency. Those factors change everything about a nurse, from the types of shoes she chooses to wear, the kinds of scrubs she buys, and how she prepares herself for a shift. For example, I used to wear hoop earrings. It was also in my first year as an ER

RN that I learned why you *shouldn't*. A drunk and violent patient tore the hoop from my ear and I required medical care.

One day, a doctor sent me to the supply closet to retrieve an item. I can't even remember what it was that I was looking for, but I do know that I couldn't find it and I was in tears because the doctor seemed to hate me. He yelled at me constantly and often told me (in front of peers and patients) that I should quit and save everyone time. One time, he told me I should kill myself because I documented on the wrong chart. I was so afraid of coming back empty-handed to this doctor, so I was a disaster.

The intercom announced a code on one of my patients, so I panicked and rushed out of the room. I was running so hard and so fast that I didn't even feel my scrub pants falling. I was two doors away from my patient's room, when my pants fell to my knees. I tripped and fell against a cart in the hallway. Half-filled cups of cold coffee and water spilled all over my blouse and skin as I lay on the hallway floor.

I managed to pull up my pants and realized that I'd lost one of my shoes in the fall. As I went to pick it up, all I could hear were the snickers of the patients and staff who'd seen what had happened.

"You're going to clean all that up," someone said to me.

Tears were streaming down my face, and all I could think about was taking off my scrub top and going to the bathroom to clean up. I figured I could change and grab a mop while I was at it.

I pulled off my top and didn't think much of it because I always wear a bra and a camisole tank top under my top.

You know, I don't know if I just wasn't paying attention or what, but when I pulled off my blouse, half my tank top was pulled down, and my right boob was hanging out of my bra.

A lot of people laughed some more.

I ran out of the ER like embarrassed teens do in movies.

That's not all.

The code?

The code wasn't real! One of doctors (the mean one) and a group of snotty nurses thought it would be 'funny' to call the code, to see how I'd react.

I called off work for three days straight, before HR called me in for an investigation. I really thought I was going to be fired, but the meeting wasn't about me. Much to my surprise, the hospital fired the nurses involved in calling the code, and they terminated their contract with the doctor. They wanted to make sure I wouldn't sue the hospital for the behavior of my peers.

I guess that group of nurses and the doctor controlled the rest of the ER staff, because once they were gone, life was much easier. The rest of that first year was still horrible, but it was a relief to finally have friends to turn to during that time.

I can sure laugh about it now, but it took a while to get to that point.

--K.L.T.
Maine

I'm Free, Free-Floating

I'm chronically ill, with a few conditions that have left me with chronic pain and fatigue. I've dealt with this since I was a kid, and finally, at the age of 15, I was diagnosed with Fibromyalgia. This diagnosis has a tendency to make medical professionals think patients are faking everything, which I've found to be especially true in the ED. Because of this, and the rest of my medical diagnosis list—not to mention that my name is listed in the state opioid database (a database that logs a patient's every prescription for Schedule II-IV medication)—I try to avoid the ED unless I think something is really wrong, just to save myself from feeling judged and disbelieved. Still, I register in the ED an average of two to three times per year. My conditions make ED trips necessary.

Several years ago, I was experiencing unbearable pain. I recognized the pain from a past experience and tried treating myself with a method that had helped alleviate the pain before. Unfortunately, this wasn't helping, so I finally gave in and agreed to let my husband take me to the ED. It was a smart decision, because it turned out I had a badly infected gallbladder, with a large gallstone blocking my bile duct. I went to emergency surgery.

Years later, I visited my doctor, and I was sent to the ED for stat blood work and a CT. I ended up in the same ED, this time registered for an ongoing GI issue.

After a moderate wait, the very seasoned ED doctor came back to my room and said, "Well, I saw something today on your scan that I've never seen before."

I can't tell you the kind of concern that's generated when a doctor—and particularly an ED doctor who's been around for a while—says that. My husband and I exchanged worried glances.

Steeling myself for bad news, I replied, "Oh?"

"You had your gallbladder removed, about, what, five years ago?" he asked, as he settled onto a stool.

I nodded.

He said, "I checked the images from that ultrasound, and you have a gallstone in the same spot on your CT scan that you did from the ultrasound."

I was confused and said, "Um, what?"

Apparently, when they sucked my gallbladder out years before, the original stone that had caused so many of the issues slid out and remained in abdomen. I have a free-floating gallstone.

This isn't the first time I've had something medically-odd about me—I'm known to my friends and doctors as a bit of a medical mystery—so this was just one more oddity.

My friends took the idea and ran with it, so now my free-floating gallstone has a name: Roswell.

--T.G.

California

<u>Empathy</u>

(Author's note: This story was submitted by the author of the previous submission.)

Now that you are aware of some of my conditions, I'll share another story that isn't a funny one.

Several months ago, I was in a great deal of pain, stemming from my tooth. I had a dentist appointment coming up, had a supply of OraGel on hand, and had no desire to face another medical bill. I tried so hard to avoid seeking medical attention, but about one in the morning, the pain was so severe that I couldn't stand it any longer. I had nerve pain shooting up and down the right side of my face.

Now, I deal with neuropathy, joint hypermobility, and something on the autoimmune spectrum. I am on a whole host of medications to help keep me as healthy as I can bed and avoid more organ, joint, and tissue damage. My 'normal' pain level at the time was between a six and seven—and that was considered a good day. Like many chronic pain patients, I show very little outward signs that I am in pain, and I tend to use humor to diffuse situations. I tried treating myself with dental products and by taking a dose of Percocet, just one of many medications I've had ordered to me routinely. This night, though, OraGel and Percocet couldn't offer even an ounce of relief, and I was close to screaming. Given my other health issues, I became concerned that there was something terribly wrong, something more than just a tooth in need of a root canal.

Finally, I had to admit that I needed to seek help. Off to the ED we went.

When the doctor walked in, the first words out of her mouth were, "I'm not giving you any narcotics."

I blinked in surprise before responding, "Okay, I'm not here for narcotics. They're not working."

She sighed. Then, she asked me what my issue was. I explained that I was experiencing progressively worsening nerve pain, and with my neuropathy and other health history-and the fact that nothing could ease the pain-that I was worried.

This doctor eventually examined me, and after just *listening* to what I was saying, she exclaimed, "Oh! I think I can help you."

It was a smart move to go to the ED that night, because I had a badly infected parotid gland. After some antibiotics and a shot of Toradol to treat inflammation (even though the pain hadn't started to dissipate yet), I started to relax, knowing that the problem was being addressed.

The doctor and I were able to have a conversation about what my life with chronic pain was like, discussed the medications I've tried and failed on, talk about diagnoses I've collected over the years, the hundreds of tests I've undergone, and, most importantly, the fact that I—like the majority of chronic pain patients I know—use my prescriptions responsibly.

I'd like to think that maybe I gave her something to think about when it comes to treatment of chronic pain patients.

<u>Oops, My Bad</u>

I read about your PVC pipe story, and I have one of my own!

So, this guy came hobbling in the ED one day. He was clearly intoxicated, evident by his cherry, glossy eyes, slurred speech, and the ETOH emissions he was giving off.

This man couldn't walk normally because he had a PVC pipe around from his mid-calf to his upper thigh. He walked as if he had a peg leg because he couldn't bend his left knee.

Registration called, but our treatment rooms were filled with cardiac patients and patients displaying CVA (stroke) symptoms. We instructed the clerk to send the man to the waiting room. We could hear him hollering all the way in our break room, which was separated by a thick brick wall and two sets of glass doors. Security had to get involved.

By the time we called this man to the back, the alcohol in his system had more time to kick in, so he was combative. I don't know for sure, but I had a feeling this man was an asshole when he wasn't drunk, too. A doctor ordered restraints for this patient, after the man punched a tech.

Now, with the violent patient restrained, we were faced with the task of removing the pipe. It sure was on there tight. Doctors were afraid of using cutters to remove the piece, just because it appeared to be suctioned against his skin. We all thought the safest option would be to introduce lubricant and attempt to 'jiggle' the piece until it was loose enough to slip off or cut off.

Want to guess which nurse was assigned that task?

Who has two thumbs and absolutely *loves* being called a fat cow, when she's only trying to *help* some imbecile who thought it'd be a bright idea to stick his leg in a PVC pipe?

I first tried standing at the patient's feet, and I wrapped my hands around the pipe's center to pull downward. The pipe didn't budge, but it was worth a shot. If you asked the patient, I'm positive he would have told you otherwise. He was cursing and calling me names during my attempt.

I gave up on working from the patient's feet, so I moved toward his chest. I couldn't wait to get out of the room because this jerk was using all his energy to flop his body around like a fish out of water. He pulled at the restraints until I thought they'd break, and at one point, he headbutted me in the shoulder. It took him spitting on me for the unit clerk to finally call the police.

Honestly, and I know it was wrong of me, I started thinking that maybe we should just send the guy to jail with the pipe on his leg. He didn't seem to be appreciative of my efforts to free him. But, I started thinking of those videos my Facebook friends share. I'm sure you've seen them. There will be a video of a raccoon stuck in a fence or something, and when hikers try to free it, the raccoon snaps, and claws at its saviors. Maybe the patient was a trapped raccoon, desperate for help but still a wild animal.

I told the patient to stop moving around, but he wouldn't listen. In fact, giving him an order seemed to rile him up even more.

Finally, I just ignored his shouting and his movement, and I hovered over his chest at an angle. I pulled and pulled at that pipe, hoping to pull it up just enough to loosen from his skin. If we could move it even an inch, we figured doctors would have a small space between the pipe and skin to start cutting.

While I was using all my strength to move this pipe, the patient started in on violent threats against me. He told me he was going to rape me, said he wanted to stab me, and then started in on my appearance.

My hands slipped away from the pipe and I elbowed the patient in the nose.

I swear, it was an accident. It felt so good, though, in a way. I mean, I did feel some remorse, but the other part of me wanted to ask the patient, "What was that? Do you have anything else to say?"

I don't know if he could've answered that because he started *crying* like a big baby! Mr. Tough Guy apparently just needed to have his butt kicked, because as soon as I elbowed his nose, he was a completely different person. I didn't even break his nose!

We never could get the pipe to budge, so doctors used cutters with minimal damage to the patient's skin. The patient cried through the entire process.

I had to file statements with the police, HR, and my department, but I didn't get in trouble.

--C.T.
Arizona

<u>Well, Go Get Her!</u>

I am a Registered Sleep Technician. You are probably familiar with my common job description: I watch patients sleep and monitor brain activity, breathing patterns, and patient behavior.

I usually do not share my second most common job description: I monitor patients for impotence by verifying if the patient develops a nocturnal erection. This study is done to 'prove' impotence in men claiming they cannot achieve an erection. These patients are usually trying to figure out if they are good candidates for penile implants, or to rule out other factors, such as psychological factors. It's a largely-outdated practice, but our facility is kind of 'old school.'

Prior to the patient's 'bed time,' I affix a paper band around the patient's flaccid penis. If a patient develops and erection and the band breaks, I am to wake the patient to show him the erection. (I guess the department did not always do this, but apparently patients didn't take the staff's word for it, hence our waking policy.) Most patients eventually fall asleep after hearing the news. If the patient does not develop a nocturnal erection, I note this in the patient's chart, which is viewed by the patient's doctor.

Well, I had this patient one night, and he was probably in his late-60s. As he was preparing for the study, he told me all about how he 'needed' the implant. He and his wife had not had intercourse in more than a year, and he was 'sure' an implant could help them.

About five hours into the study, the patient achieved a nocturnal erection and his paper band broke.

I went into the bed area to awake the patient. It took at least four hard shakes to the man's shoulders (after trying softer methods) to wake him.

"Mr. Doe," I said quietly, "I'm required to wake you to show you that you achieved a nocturnal erection."

The patient's eyes popped wide open, as if I'd just told him the building was on fire, and he exclaimed, "Go get my wife. Tell her to hurry! She's getting some nookie tonight!"

I didn't have a clue in the world how to react to this, so I kind of laughed it off. The patient was serious, though. When I told him that I couldn't allow him to have sex with his wife in the sleep lab, he left AMA. All I could do was note it in his chart.

When the opportunity...ahem, arises...you just have to seize it.

--E.M.
Illinois

The Extremes We Take...

First off, I'm just going to say it, Kerry: I am an idiot. An idiot with good intentions, but an idiot nonetheless…

I was a little pudgy around the middle…and top…and bottom—okay, I was a little porky, I'll admit it. I didn't realize how much it affected me until I went to a bar after work and one of the pretty guys I asked to dance said he wasn't attracted to 'fat guys.' Yeah, ouch, that hurt. But, I decided to start dieting and exercising instead of wallowing in my sorrow.

The thing is, dieting and exercising are *hard*. Going to the gym after working 12-15-hour shifts is *really hard*. I couldn't afford a treadmill, and there was no way I could get a weight center moved up two flights of stairs to my apartment.

Well, on day three of my new diet, while I was eating a whole bag of chips (I don't have self-control, okay?!) and surfing the internet, I saw this fitness sliding board thing. What it was in the pictures was this long black plastic-ish mat that you put on the floor. The people in the pictures and videos wore these thin nylon booties, and then they stood on the mat and slid from side to side. The pictures and videos showed these people effortlessly sliding while they were grinning and talking to their workout buddies in this place that looked like a dance studio. Of course, I knew my experience would differ. I already pictured myself sweating profusely, as I slid from side to side in front of an episode of *'Sons of Anarchy.'*

The board was kind of pricey, but I figured if it really was a decent piece of low-impact fitness equipment and could help me lose about 20 pounds, it'd be worth the cost.

Thanks to my Prime account, the board arrived in two days. It was kind of hard to open the box, so as I was walking through the kitchen, I grabbed the closest sharp object I could find, which just happened to be a corkscrew. I opened the box in the living room and tossed the corkscrew to my ottoman, where it landed awkwardly on a pile of clothes.

I read the instructions and the FAQs for the board. I specifically recall reading a statement in bold that said not to put lubricant on the board, that at first it may not be as slick as I'd expect, but over time, the nylon booties would 'buff' the plastic, which would make it slicker and easier to slide.

Well, I was pumped, right? I could work out in my living room. You know what that means? It meant I didn't have to wear pants.

So, there I was, in my tighty-whities and a tank top that smelled like nachos because I pulled it out of the dirty clothes basket, and I was flipping through my list on Netflix until I found my show. I moved my ottoman back a little bit, and I put the board on the hardwood floor, between the TV stand and the ottoman. Man, this was gonna be good.

Man, it was not good.

No matter how much I tried, I couldn't really get a good 'slide' going. The board just wasn't slick enough.

Despite having read only a few minutes earlier *not* to put oil on the board, you know what I did?

Yeah, I went to the kitchen again and came back with Pam cooking spray. I didn't even spray on a little. I sprayed that thing until oil was running off the sides.

I'd read somewhere—probably in an online article or something on Pinterest—where you should exercise with weights to enhance your workout, so I grabbed my 50-pound weights from the corners and held one in each hand.

I stepped on the board and remained steady. Yeah, I was going to get sexy! I'd be so buff that I'd be like Alex on *'Grey's Anatomy,'* the kind of guy all the women at worked talked about—you know, those hot guys with pecs bursting out of their scrubs. Yep, that was going to be me.

I pushed off and to say I slid would be an understatement. Listen, if I had used anymore force, I would have flown out my damn window, I swear. The only thing stopping that from happening were the wooden buffers on each end of the board.

So, instead of flying out the window, I fell backwards. I felt a sharp pain in the back of my head, but I was too worried about still moving that I didn't have time to give it much thought. In about two more seconds, I did the splits.

I have never done the splits before that moment.

When I say I did the splits, I mean my balls were touching the ground. I somehow dropped one of the weights on my fingers and the other one hit me in the groin, which already hurt like I can't even explain. It hurt so much that I made this high-pitched squeal and puked.

I had to reach behind me for my phone and call 911 because I thought, for sure, my testicles were going to need to be amputated.

Oh my God, I'm 25 and I'm going to have to go through the rest of my life explaining that I don't have balls because I had a bad exercising accident.

I felt something trickle down the back of my neck and touched it. There was blood everywhere. I was afraid to touch my head because it hurt, and I was bleeding *a lot.*

Double 'oh my God.' I'm going to bleed out before the paramedics can even get to my apartment. They're going to find me dead on the floor, still in the splits position, wearing nothing but underwear and a dirty shirt, having bled to death.

Thankfully, the medics took about six minutes to get to my apartment. I guess they were staging a few blocks away.

The guys were sympathetic to my delicate situation. They didn't crack any jokes (but I bet they wanted to), even as I was bawling and kept puking because the pain was so bad.

My neighbors were standing in the hallway as the medics took me out on a stretcher.

The lady next door rushed up to us and asked, "What happened?"

I responded in a frantic scream that rang throughout the building, "I lost my balls, Deborah!"

You know, my workplace has all these mandatory training seminars and sends 20,000 emails about HIPAA, but when you work at the same ER that the medics take you to, forget about HIPAA. I had to see *every-single-one* of my coworkers while I was admitted. They just 'popped in to say hi' and 'check on' me. I've always kept a mental list of doctors I *didn't* want to work on me if I was ever a patient, but at that point, you could have sent Scooby-Doo wearing a lab coat in to see me, and I would have been grateful.

I calmed down after some Dilaudid (now I know why so many people come in for it), and a piggy back of Zofran stopped my vomiting.

I sustained what the doctors called a 'small' tear to my scrotum and received eight sutures. There was concern of a severe testicular rupture, but the swelling was determined to be a minor result of the splits, hitting the floor, and hitting myself with the weight. Additionally, I sustained two broken fingers. The corkscrew was still stuck in my head upon examination, but after a few minutes of applying pressure, the wound clotted on its own.

I returned home with swollen balls, broken fingers, and a bruised head. The doctor gave me a work-release for five days, and I needed all five days to sit on my couch with an ice pack to my groin.

I threw that board out. If I'm fat, I'm fat, okay? If God wanted me to look like Hercules, he would have given me the genetics to be able to eat anything I want and gain muscle definition by lifting my TV remote. Nursing is my cardio.

--T.J.
New York

<u>Awkward</u>

I work on a floor where patients have limited mobility. It's my job to help patients to the restroom, to bathe patients (either in bed or in the tub), feed patients, and generally assist them with anything they cannot do for themselves. I wouldn't say my job is glamorous by any means, but I am proud of what I do. Even on the bad days, I realize my life could be a lot worse.

I was assigned to a middle-age woman, Jane, who'd recently been paralyzed from the neck down. She was left in a state of severe mental decline. She could no longer speak coherently, and she would be considered disabled for the rest of her life. Her orders required a light bedside bath (or what most would consider a 'sponge bath'), due to recent surgeries.

Jane's husband was in the room when I arrived. I introduced myself and explained that I was there to bathe the patient. This man seemed 'normal,' and told me he'd like to stay in the room because he was watching a baseball game and didn't want to miss the last inning. I did not see anything wrong with this.

I filled my 'bath tote' with warm water from the bathroom and placed it on a cart. I faced away from the patient's husband and opened the patient's gown. I spoke to her as I bathed her, explaining which body part I was washing, and I also talked about the weather, the art on the wall, and generally tried to keep talking because I feel it's important that the patient feels that I care, not that I'm just there to treat them like a bump on a log. I heard Jane's husband making some grunting noises from behind me, but my grandfather is old and makes the same noises when he's watching the news or football, so I just figured the man was mad about the ball game.

As I was moving my cart to the other side of the bed, I just happened to look over to Jane's husband.

You wouldn't freaking believe it.

This man had his jeans unzipped and was masturbating while staring at me.

I exclaimed in shock and he said breathily, "Don't stop now, honey. Why don't you bend over for me again? Let me see that ass."

I ran out of the room and called my supervisor and security. They confronted the patient's husband and he admitted to masturbating while I was in the room. My superiors called the police department and the man was arrested for exposing himself and lewd behavior.

I don't know what happened to the patient's husband because that day was my last before my vacation, and by the time I'd come back to work, Jane had been transferred to an assisted living facility.

To this day, my skin crawls when I hear my grandpa making those grunting noises. I actually have to leave the room or interrupt him because all I can think of is Jane's husband.

--O.L.
Washington

A Simple Mistake

My contract for ES physician with another hospital ended, and instead of renewing it, I transferred to a facility in another state.

I had practiced at my previous facility for close to a decade, so I had become quite familiar with the hospital's layout. I was lost, to say the least, for a while in the new hospital.

One thing I just couldn't get accustomed to was the location of hand sanitizer dispensers.

At the old place, the dispensers were on the right when you entered the patient's room. That makes sense, right? You walk in, stick out your right hand, and there's the sanitizer.

At this new place, it was, 'Okay, we'll set you loose, and good luck finding the dispensers.' In some rooms, the dispensers would be by the sink, while in other rooms, the dispensers would be on the wall behind the bed. It made no sense to me.

Now that I've filled you in, I'll tell you about my embarrassing moment.

I entered a patient's room and proceeded to conduct an examination. The patient jabbered about how he only believed in holistic medicine, and how he did not believe I knew what I was talking about. I did not take it personally.

About halfway through, I sat down and told the man the truth, which was, "You can try alternative medicine if you'd like, but you're more likely to die before it helps you. Or, you can take this medication, have the surgery, and you should go on to live a long, happy life."

The patient still didn't want to hear anything I had to say. Some days, I'm convinced these people pay thousands of dollars to the ES on the slight chance that a healthcare professional will tell them what they want to hear. I don't know if it's out of ego, fear, or maybe a combination of the two, but I'm not in the business of telling anyone what they *want* to hear; I'm in the business of telling folks what they *need* to hear.

With the patient's interest fading and his attitude growing, I decided that was enough. I'd laid out his options, so he could take it from there. I looked around for a second and found the hand sanitizer dispenser, and I pumped a glob of the white foam on my palm. I was going to leave as soon as I finished rubbing the stuff into my skin. Mentally, I was trying to remember our conversation verbatim, so I could chart properly.

After a few seconds of mindlessly rubbing, I realized the sanitizer was not drying.

I rubbed a bit harder and tried to spread some of it up my forearms.

The patient scoffed and said, as he shook his head, "You do know that's soap, right?"

Damn.

He walked out, muttering along the way, "And this idiot thinks he knows it all."

Well, I lost all credibility with that patient, but I can tell you I never made that mistake again. I'm so incredibly glad that I spent $200,000 on tuition and supplies, with years spent studying and shadowing an endless number of fellow physicians, only to not realize I was smearing hand soap all over my hands and arms. I might just be genius material.

--V.S., M.D.
Florida

<u>Scenic Route</u>

I had been retired from EMS for about ten years on the day I was driving through what I like to call 'The Void.' This area is nothing but fields for miles and miles. There are no houses, abandoned barns, or any other structures in sight. If you're driving through The Void, you'd sure better have some good music to keep you awake, because it can be a boring drive.

Maybe halfway through The Void, when I was about, say 30-40 miles in, I thought I saw a naked man ahead. I blinked a few times. Surely, I was just exhausted from driving back from California, where I had attended my father's funeral. There couldn't be a naked man ahead. There just couldn't be.

There was.

This man was tall and lanky, with sunken eyes and craters on his face. He looked like a dead man walking, honestly.

And then he jumped out in front of my car.

Luckily, I had slowed down when I had first noticed him, so I didn't hit him.

He ran to my passenger door and pulled on the handle. My doors automatically lock when I am traveling, so thank goodness for that.

"Let me in!" he screamed. "You have to let me in! They're going to get me!"

I rolled the window down just enough to try to figure out what the heck was going on.

"Are you in danger?" I asked.

"We're all in danger!" he yelled with a screech that scared off a flock of turkey vultures near the tree line across the single-lane road.

"Are you on something?" I asked.

He violently shook his head. "You gotta let me in. We gotta go. I ain't on nothing. But we gotta go. Like, right now."

The medic in me came out, so I blurted, "If you're not on anything, then why in God's name are you naked in the middle of nowhere?"

He pointed to a cornfield about a mile away and said, "They're in there. And they're after me."

"What is?" I asked.

"Not what," he whispered dramatically. "Who."

Here's something that happens in the medical field that not many people know happens. I'm sure you know all about it. See, when working in the medical field, one often comes across the stupidest, craziest patients. And, since it's 'unprofessional' or 'socially unacceptable' to call someone out for this or to generally react in any way other than worshipping the ground these wacko patients walk on (which I find absolutely ludicrous— maybe if we start telling these people how stupid they are, we won't be letting someone with chest pains die while we're responding to a call of dental pain at 03:00), many of us have developed what I call, 'The Internal Eyeroll.' This is when you can be looking a patient dead in the eyes and your outer appearance remains unaffected, but it's almost as if you have a second pair of eyeballs behind those, and you roll them so hard you can actually feel them falling out the back of your skull. The Internal Eyeroll is oft accompanied by thoughts you shouldn't say aloud.

But, since I was retired, I could say whatever I wanted.

"You really think someone would be after you, when you look like a tweeking skeleton?" I asked.

The man started pulling on my door handle again, with no regard to my question. He begged for me to let him in and take him far away.

It was clear someone needed to intervene. What if I drove away, but a young mother or an elderly woman drove by next and saw the man? If they didn't have their car doors locked, or if they got out of their vehicles to help the man, there was no telling what would happen.

My cell phone did not receive service in The Void, but luckily, I still had my CB installed. I didn't know if I could find a channel that police monitored, so I tried a few calling out a few times, before a man with a gruff voice answered. He said he was a trucker and he was on the other side of The Void, traveling on a highway. I gave him my location and asked him to call authorities.

"You wreck or something?" he asked.

"Or something," I said.

"Now," I said to the naked man, who was just as frantic all this time later, "I've called the police. They're on their way."

"You what?!" he screamed. "You shouldn't have done that. Don't you know they're in on it?"

For a good hour, the naked man circled my vehicle and tried to get in every door. At one point, he even tried to elbow my back windshield. He must've hurt himself pretty good, because he rolled around on the asphalt for a little bit, before getting right back up and trying to get in my car again.

When I could finally see a patrol car in my rearview mirror, the naked man threw himself on the hood of my car and started punching my windshield until his knuckles bled.

I still didn't get out of my vehicle, but two officers got out of their patrol car. They attempted to calm the naked man by speaking to him, but that got them nowhere. When they tried to place them under arrest, he spit on one officer and took off running. Picture it: Skeletor, in late-summer, running alongside a country road, completely naked.

One officer chased the man, while the other officer followed in the patrol car.

It didn't end well for the man. The officer on-foot tased the subject, and this guy hit the ground in about two-seconds flat.

After officers handcuffed and 'tucked away' (put him in the back of the patrol car) the man, I got out of my car.

"He's definitely on something," one of the officers told me. He pointed to where the man was tased and said, "He was just telling me he's being chased by those Stephen King things."

"The clown?" his partner asked.

"No," the first officer replied. "Those kids in the corn."

I couldn't help but to laugh.

None of us could figure out where the man came from or why he was naked, but drugs were the probable cause. It wouldn't surprise me if the man had some mental problems as well.

Now, I don't know what happened to this man, because I live in the next county and don't get news from The Void or its county, but I do know the man busted up my windshield enough that I had to pay a $400 deductible, on top of the hassle of being without a vehicle while mine was in the shop.

-L.W.
Iowa

<u>Holy Moly</u>

I can't recall why my patient was going to surgery, but I do know it was my job to enter his room and prepare him for the procedure. I was ordered to shave the patient's groin.

I entered the room with my supplies. The patient was in his late-20s. A young woman, maybe in her mid-20s, was sitting at the patient's bedside. She was playing with her phone, but as soon as I came in, she put the phone down and started giving me dirty looks. At first, I didn't know why.

I introduced myself to the patient and explained the shaving process, assuring him that I practiced the utmost care when caring for my patients. He seemed to understand.

"So, wait," the young woman said. "You're going to be touching his dick?"

"This is a pre-operative measure," I explained. "You don't have to stay in the room if this isn't comfortable for you."

I then looked to the patient and said, "And you are more than welcome to ask your company to leave, if you would like me to do this in private."

"Uh, I'm his girlfriend," the woman said loudly.

I looked at this girl blankly and said, "Okay..."

"So, why are you coming in here to grab my boyfriend's dick?" she shouted.

"Uh," I said, "I'm here to shave him. It's standard pre-op procedure."

"Yeah, right," the woman said. "I'm sure you saw him and just couldn't wait to get your hands on him. You're a slut."

She said that with a few more curse words, but the message was just the same.

"Babe," the guy said, "calm down."

Telling a woman to 'calm down' almost guarantees that she will do anything *but*.

She flung her arms out to her sides and screamed, "Oh, so now you *want* some other girl to touch your dick? You're going to cheat on me, while I'm in the room? You're going to let this whore jerk you off?"

"Ma'am," I said firmly, but calmly, "I'm going to need you to leave the room."

"I am his girlfriend," the woman yelled slowly, talking to me like I was stupid.

"And I understand that, but I have a job to do. You're interfering. If your boyfriend doesn't have this done, he won't be able to go to surgery."

"I don't care," she shrugged. "I'm not going to sit in here and let some slut grab his dick."

I sighed and looked away at my imaginary camera crew, before I started to walk away.

"Yeah, you'd better run, bitch," the woman shouted. "You're a whore!"

"You are so crazy," said the patient.

"Don't do that. Don't call me crazy and try to make me think I'm imagining stuff, when you're *clearly* okay with having some other slut grab your dick. You're gaslighting me. I'm your girlfriend. I should be the only person near you like that."

"She's a nurse!" the patient exclaimed.

"And?"

"It's her job!"

"So, what you're saying, is that it's okay to cheat, just because she's a nurse?"

"Oh my God," the patient groaned. "You are so freaking crazy."

"Hey," the patient called to me, "don't go. Please? I really need this surgery."

"Oh, I can't believe you!" the woman shrieked. "I can't even believe you!"

I turned to the patient and stated, "Sir, I will be right back."

"Like hell you will," the woman said. "If you come back in here, I swear, I'm going to beat your ass."

"Okay," I said, shrugging. "We'll see about that."

This woman was my age. I couldn't believe she was acting this way and over something like shaving a man's groin! Did she really think I would be holding her man's flaccid penis in my gloved hand and suddenly get the urge to take off my clothes and tell him to take me? Come on, now. I am not remotely interested in sex with patients. I am in so much debt from student loans and credit cards that I'm not remotely interested in *any* man, at least until I can dig myself out of this hole. I have enough stress in my life just from comparing my budget to my bills; I certainly don't need to concern myself with trying to budget in birthday gifts, dinners, and birth control, just to have a relationship. I'm fine with my cat and Hulu subscription, thank you very much. (Author's note: AMEN.)

With this woman still yelling and threatening me, I left the room. I couldn't find any of the unit nurses, so I walked over to a phone and dialed security. I was so done with this woman's attitude, that I was about to show her mine. Seriously, what would possess someone to enter a hospital and think they could get away with that type of behavior? My only guess is that, if she displayed that behavior elsewhere, the staff let it slide to avoid negative facility feedback, or to avoid the drama. But, if you're going to try to prevent me from doing my job…the job that doesn't even begin to pay me enough to put up with crap like that…you'd better believe that I'm going to handle the problem.

The woman was still shouting at her boyfriend and me when two security guards arrived. I didn't have to explain the situation to the guards, because the woman was acting like such a horse's ass that they could figure it all out on their own.

Security entered the room first, and I stood behind them and in a corner, near my supply cart.

"You are such a stupid slut," the woman yelled. "You think that some rent-a-cops are going to be able to save you?"

This woman then picked up the lamp at her boyfriend's bedside, and she threw it at me. I dodged the lamp and it broke as soon as it hit the wall.

Security tried to remove the woman without force, but she assaulted both men. That's when they wrestled her to the ground. She was still fighting, spitting, and screaming when they cuffed her. One guard used his radio to ask someone to call the police. They took the woman to the hallway. I don't think she went a full thirty seconds in silence. The whole time, the patient was shaking his head and muttering to himself. He apologized to me a few times.

The woman in the hallway threatened that she was going to 'track me down' and beat me so badly that I would be a patient at the hospital. That's a really stupid thing to say to a nurse in front of witnesses, by the way. When the cops arrived, the woman was arrested. I had to give a statement and sign paperwork. The woman's boyfriend said she had just moved in with him last week, but he asked me if he could use a phone to call his mother. He wanted someone from his family to go to his apartment and pack up all the woman's stuff. He said he was so embarrassed by her behavior and that this moment made him realize he didn't want to spend another minute with her. He then asked me if we could place her on the no-visit list. It was my pleasure to add her list to the restricted visitor list.

I couldn't shave the patient for about an hour after I initially entered the room and this mess started, but when I did, the procedure took about 10 minutes, and then I never saw him again. All that fuss over nothing!

I *did* see the patient's ex-girlfriend again. She somehow found me from a public Facebook post the hospital made. I had 'liked' the post, so she then had my full name and a link to my personal profile. I guess she went through all the hospital's posts and clicked on profiles until she found mine. She started spam-messaging me with threats, so I blocked her from contacting me—online, at least. The woman was in the parking lot as I was leaving one night, and I called security. She was arrested, but she didn't do any serious time because her judge said that what she was doing wasn't felony stalking. I filed for a restraining order, and I never saw her again.

Without a doubt, this was the craziest thing I've ever experienced at work.

--G.K.
Ohio

One Big Happy Family

A mother rushed to our triage nurse during our evening shift change, pleading and screaming for us to help her son. Six children ranging from 5 to 15 followed her.

"What happened?" the triage nurse asked.

"They were all jumping on the trampoline. He fell off and won't wake up."

"Go over to her," triage said, as she pointed to me. "Tell her your son's name and birthday. I'll take him to the back, and then she'll bring you back with us. Jane, find us in room eight."

I nodded.

The woman sprinted to my desk and said, "His name is John Smith."

"Mom," one of the boys said.

"Not now."

"But mom," the child nagged.

"Not now, Joe!"

I quickly entered the patient in the computer and took the family back to room eight, where there were tons of people huddle around the injured boy. One doctor got flustered with so many kids in the room and yelled, "Can someone take all these kids to the cafeteria or something?"

Two techs volunteered and took the other kids out of the room. I went back up front.

About five minutes later, the mother came barreling out of the emergency room, crying so hard I could barely understand her. I started thinking she was given bad news about her son's condition.

"I messed up," she said to me.

"It's okay," I said, trying to keep her from blowing snot at me as she tried to breathe.

"It's not okay," she cried. "I'm a horrible mother."

"Accidents happen all the time," I assured her. "Kids fall. That's what they do."

She stopped crying and looked at me, confused.

"No," she said. "I gave you the wrong name."

"Huh?"

"That's not John back there. That's Joe. I got my kids mixed up."

"Well," I reasoned, "that can happen with twins."

The woman started sobbing again and said, "That's just it. They're not twins! They're two years apart!"

We had to call our software provider to remove the information charted to the wrong patient's chart, and we had to re-register the correct patient and play catch-up to add the correct charges and details to his chart.

The kid turned out to be okay, for the most part. He did have a small crack in his skull and they said he cracked a rib, but he was discharged after a few hours.

--P.R.
Texas

Up a Tree

We (at the fire station) received a direct call from a concerned citizen, reporting a cat stuck in a tree. Generally, we attempt to convince the citizen that cats do not remain 'stuck' in trees, but to ease their minds, we take the cat's location and tell the caller that we will do a routine drive-by after a few hours. (We actually do perform the drive-by, just in case. This is not something we tell callers to get them off our backs.)

In this case, we were informed that the cat was not alone in the tree. There was also a middle-age male in the tree, claiming he was stuck and could not get down. We notified dispatch and left the station.

We arrived on scene only minutes following the call. Indeed, about halfway up this 40 to 50-foot tree, was a middle age male, who was screaming at concerned onlookers. I guess I should paint a better picture here.

This tree has been on our town's square for as long as I remember, and I was 65 at the time. It's really a beautiful tree, with small flowers that bud during Spring. It rests on the courthouse lawn and overlooks our small town, which has a population of roughly 1,200. This incident occurred on Homecoming weekend, so most of the 1,200 people from our town were on the square. I'd say about 400 people were around this tree or nearby, at least, to watch this fool.

Now, I say this man is a fool because he was clutching Jane Smith's cat. We know this was Jane Smith's cat, because he's worn the same blue collar for eight years, and he's a climber. We chase him off our ladders at least twice a week, and we've seen him in every tree in town. The cat was in no danger of being 'stuck,' except it kind of was 'stuck,' since the town drunk was holding it hostage.

The man was yelling for someone to help him.

"Let go of the cat," I yelled.

"I can't. If I let him go, he won't be able to get down."

"John," I hollered to the man, as the cat was scratching him to hell, "let go of the cat.

He doesn't want you holding him. Just let him go, and he'll come down on his own."

John argued with me for a good five minutes, before the cat bit him and John finally released the cat.

We tried to move the crowd out of the way, so we could move in closer to raise the ladder and help John out of the tree.

"I am so drunk right now," John called to me. "I think I'm going to puke."

"We're going to get you down, buddy," I called.

"Am I going to jail?" he asked.

I replied honestly and said, "You're probably going to be in some trouble, yeah."

"Then go away," he said. "I'm not coming down."

"John," I sighed, "don't worry about that right now. We need to get you down from there."

"No," he said, "I'm going to stay up here. You can go."

"You're going to fall," I said. "Just let us help you down, and we'll worry about the rest when you're safe."

"I'm not gonna fall," John said—right before he fell.

The crowd screamed, and we rushed in. John had fallen about 20-25 feet. He appeared lifeless as we approached him, and his neck was in an unnatural position.

After a quick assessment, we realized John was still breathing.

We called out for an ambulance, which took longer to arrive because our town only has one ambulance—which was across town, at the park, in the parade lineup.

John was transported to the nearest hospital, which is about 30-minutes away. He suffered a broken neck, but otherwise, he was fine. He was court-ordered to a rehab facility for 30 days, and he was ordered to attend alcohol dependence support groups for one year. I'm sad to report that John violated his court order by drinking as soon as he returned from rehab. He's been in and out of trouble since returning, but I can report that he has not climbed a tree since that day.

On a side note, following John's accident, our town voted to purchase a second ambulance.

--P.W.

Montana

Now You Know

At approximately 19:00 on a quiet weekday, a frantic woman called our ER and told us that she found her adult son passed out on his bedroom floor. She could not tell if he was breathing, but she stated he was bleeding from a head laceration, which appeared to be caused by a broken lamp under and beside him. He apparently fell and broke the lamp on his way down.

Our Charge instructed the woman to call 911.

Minutes later, EMS radioed a report of the patient in transport. The male was in his late-teens, and he was displaying shallow breathing, weak pulse, and his blood pressure was reading at an astronomically low number. Medics stated the patient was unconscious.

When the patient arrived at our ER, we were already waiting for him. We did not know what we were dealing with in terms of what caused the patient's condition, so we tried to stabilize his vitals and ran first-priority blood work.

While some of us were working on the patient, I went to the lobby to meet his mother. She was hysterical, and it took five minutes to calm her down enough to answer questions.

When I asked if her son was a user of tobacco, alcohol, and/or illegal/recreational drugs, she stated that he did drink, but he'd never smoked. She did not *think* he used drugs, but she said she could not rule it out. She stated she did not see evidence of drugs near or on his person when she found him in his bedroom, but he did have a glass of what appeared to be Jack Daniels on his computer desk. She knew he'd just purchased the bottle that morning, and it appeared that only one to two glasses had been poured.

Mentally, I was ruling out alcohol poisoning as the source of the patient's condition, just because when we receive patients presenting with that, they are usually semi-lucid, often are covered in vomit or are actively vomiting, and they usually reek of alcohol. Our patient presented none of these typical indicators.

Charge came to the front and motioned for me to come with her. I excused myself from the patient's mother and told her we would keep her updated. For the time, we did not think allowing her to visit would be a good idea, simply due to the number of staff in and out of her son's room.

I stood outside the patient's room with Charge, who informed me the patient was coming in and out of consciousness. She wanted me to stay with the patient and attempt to get any information from him that I could. Unfortunately, the attention he had been receiving needed to go to two children who'd been found unresponsive in a swimming pool. This was not a case of 'a child's life is more important,' but a case of, 'we've managed to stabilize this patient for now, and we've done all we can do until his lab results are back.'

I felt useless as I remained at the patient's bedside. While my coworkers were preparing for the incoming drowning victims, I was sitting in an uncomfortable chair, staring at my patient, hoping he'd wake up.

EMS rushed in two toddlers. I could hear their parents screaming and crying from the lobby. We generally allow parents in the back, but in situations such as this, we ask that parents stay in the lobby while we transfer the patient(s) to a bed and start stabilization. I watched as EMS moved out of the way and the parents were brought back. They were crying. Their only children, twins, somehow escaped from the house while the mother was cooking dinner, and their father found them in the pool when he went to take the trash to the curb. They had last been seen approximately six to ten minutes earlier, and doctors suggested the children had been in the water for three to four minutes. I so badly wanted to be there to help, to hold the mother as she screamed, to *do something*.

My patient stirred. He opened his eyes ever-so-slightly.

"Mr. Smith? Can you hear me?"

He closed his eyes again and I gently shook his shoulder.

"John," I said, "you're at the hospital. I need you to stay awake and talk to me. Can you do that, John?"

He opened his eyes again and moved his eyeballs slowly, taking in his surroundings.

"Did you ingest anything?" I asked.

I had to keep shaking his shoulder to keep him focused.

"John, did you ingest anything? Come on, I need you to stay awake to answer this question. We're trying to help you, but we can't right now."

He struggled to lift his arm and groaned when he couldn't. Instead, he weakly pointed his index finger to the ceiling.

"I need you to answer me," I said, growing frustrated. "John, I need you to tell me if you took anything."

He pointed to the ceiling again.

"The lights?" I asked. "We know, you hit your head on the lamp. Don't worry about that, it was just a scratch."

He tried to shake his head and pointed upward.

"John," I said, "I don't know what that means. Can you speak right now? Do you think you can tell me what you took?"

After a great deal of stuttering, he managed to say, "Pocket."

Immediately, I sprung into action and began patting at John's jean pockets. Finally, in one of the cargo pockets, I found a small baggy of small white tablets, single-scored on one side (a single 'line' or indention on the pill). Upon initial investigation, one might believe these tablets to be aspirin. The two drugs are almost the same size, with similar texture. However, with closer examination, I properly identified this drug. The patient was carrying a baggy filled with Rohypnol. This drug is most commonly known as the 'roofie,' or 'date rape drug.'

I tracked down a doctor and explained the situation. We immediately started the patient on Flumazenil to counteract the drug's effect on the patient. We also were required to notify law enforcement, because Rohypnol is an illegal substance, and our patient was in possession of approximately 20 tablets.

As the patient came down from his high, he began panicking about our notifying law enforcement. We tried to keep him calm because his vitals were still a mess, but he was crying, vomiting, and pleading for us to call the cops back to tell them we had made a mistake in identifying the drugs.

While we waited for officers to arrive, which seemed to be taking *forever*, we allowed the patient's mother back to visit her son. As soon as she found out he was likely going to jail after a night of observation, she also broke down.

Officers arrived and instructed the patient's mother to wait in the hall. I was in the room as the patient stated he purchased the drugs from someone in the neighborhood. He stated he purchased the pills to use on women who turned him down in the past, but he needed to see how long it would take for the drugs to act, so he dropped one in his own drink. When he did not feel the drug in his system, he added more and more tablets to his drink.

What the patient did not know is that Rohypnol does not work immediately. One tablet usually takes about 20 to 30 minutes to 'kick in.' The patient consumed four pills in 15 minutes, by adding them to two alcoholic beverages. Mixing this drug with alcohol strengthens its effects. Our patient basically knocked himself out.

You would think that story in itself would be enough drama, but when the patient's mother heard his confession, she stormed in the room and started slapping him. She even hit him with his call button pad. Officers tried to remove the patient's mother from the room, but she then became combative against officers. She was eventually removed from the room and handcuffed. After some time, she calmed down and tearfully apologized to the officers. I think they understood her frustration and decided not to arrest or cite her.

The patient was sick as a dog during the rest of his time in our ER. We transferred him upstairs for overnight observation, where an officer sat bedside and transported him to jail following discharge.

After we learned what the patient had done, it was difficult to feel sorry for him. By the way, the toddlers from the drowning accident both lived. They were transferred out to a pediatric hospital a few hours away, but they were both fine. Their parents brought

them in to visit us a few weeks after the
incident.

--E.N.
Illinois

We couldn't figure out why the coffee our intern made was so freaking disgusting.

One day, I followed her to the break room and asked her to make a pot, while I pretended to clean the counters.

She added 24 tablespoons of coffee to a 12-cup pot.

She admitted she had no idea what she was doing, but she thought 'the rule' was two tablespoons to each cup.

I showed her how to make it the right way…the way that wouldn't make your heart explode if you could stomach a single cup.

--T.L.
Ohio

A Not-So-Great Escape

At the time, I was employed as a medic in a large metropolitan area. On average, I'd say we made about 40-50 runs during a 12-hour shift. However, on a bad day, which is definitely what this was, our runs were almost doubled.

My partner and I had just transported a syncope pregnant woman to her preferred facility. This run had gone much like the 30 or so we'd already run in 5 hours. ER staff and EMS were getting into it left and right, and our respective employees were so stressed out that we were also turning on each other. We tried to take deep breaths, hoping that tomorrow would return to normal, but it was hard to even find time to breathe. As soon as we dropped off the pregnant woman, we were being dispatched to a suspected heart attack a few blocks away.

Traffic was crazy that day, so I remember how excited I was not to be driving. The thing about this is, that while I was avoiding road rage, I was the medic in the back of the rig…with patients. And, Lord, had the patients been testing me that day.

I groaned when we arrived on scene. I wasn't a bit fazed by the patient's condition. See, I groaned because the patient was homeless, and it was obvious he had not been to a shelter in months. I am not exaggerating this point: we could smell the patient at the curb, when he was slumped against a building in the middle of a very long alley.

We assessed the patient's condition and got him in the back of the rig. We got him hooked up to leads and attached a pulse-ox. He was in and out of consciousness and we already knew it was questionable if he would survive the trip to the hospital.

Most people outside of healthcare think we are horrible for having these thoughts, but I don't care. Come work even a day in my rig, and you'll go home thanking God you don't have to do my job day in and day out.

Look, this patient reeked. I could distinctly detect urine, feces, infection (I suspected the patient had untreated diabetic ulcers, judging by the odor), and general body odor. I could see lice moving freely through his matted hair, and he had bugs crawling on his clothes.

I found it hard to breathe and spent my time in the back just gagging and swallowing the slivers of vomit that kept creeping up my throat. Yes, I felt badly for him and wondered what kind of life he had to end up this way, but all I really cared about after about thirty seconds was getting the hell out of that rig. I yelled for my partner to 'punch it,' which is our code for 'OMG, I can't take it anymore,' and that was about a minute after we'd been moving.

I was in the back of the rig for seven minutes before we pulled in the lot. As soon as my partner threw us in park, I scrambled for the doors.

Well, I had been in such a hurry to get the hell out of there, that I somehow got my feet all tangled in cords. When I opened the doors, I tripped over all the cords.

Maybe—*maybe*—this would have been an uneventful story, had I caught myself from falling, or if I had tripped and landed on my palms.

I fell out of the rig, with cords around my ankles and boots, and the crown of my head hit the ambulance bay floor. As the world around me started going dark, I swung back, and my face smashed against the rig's grated bumper.

My partner called for help and ER staff did a quick assessment.

Get this, though: I was deemed 'probably fine,' so my boss told me to stay in service because we were so busy. I was sore and dizzy the rest of the day, and I had a cut on my cheek, but I guess I survived.

--R.Y.
New York

<u>Kinky</u>

We went on a run to a university during Spring Break. A fire alarm had been activated.

We contacted the R.A. and determined that the wing in which the alarm was activated was vacant, except for one room registered to two females. The R.A. said he knew one of the females left for Cancun, so only one female was in the room.

After we secured the wing, the R.A. escorted us to the female's dorm room. We could hear a female sobbing, and it sounded like she had been injured.

I knocked on the door and was greeted by a male. He was nude, except for holding a hand towel over his groin. He had blue and red splotches all over his chest, but I couldn't figure out what the splotches were.

"It was an accident, I swear," he said hurriedly.

"I have to respond during fire alarms," the R.A. explained to the male. "I need to talk to Jane. She's gonna have to sign a statement, so I can turn it in to administration tomorrow."

"I'm not signing anything!" a female screamed from the closet.

I peeked inside and saw a naked female standing just inside the closet, inspecting herself in a tall mirror.

We couldn't get anything out of her, but the male explained that the two had wanted to try using hot wax during sex. Since candles were banned in dorm rooms, the couple had the bright idea to melt crayons with a long-barreled BBQ lighter.

This went according to plan until the female accidentally lit her hair on fire. Her hair products acted as accelerants, and half of her hair burned off before the two could put the fire out.

I'm not even joking, this girl's hair was probably down to the middle of her back on one side, and it was just inches long on the other side, with a few random strands of hair here and there. It looked like she'd gone to a salon for a full head-shave, only to be interrupted during her appointment.

The female argued with the R.A. for a while and refused to give him a statement because she didn't want everyone to know what happened.

The next morning, the college called us and requested a copy of our report, so they found out anyway.

--R.M.
Florida

So Fresh

I worked in an assisted living facility as an aide, and I was primarily responsible for assisting patients with their hygienic needs. My patients' ages ranged drastically. My youngest patient was 32, while my oldest patient was 81. Most of the younger patients were not in the facility long-term, only until they felt comfortable and able to handle their conditions.

That day, I think I'd bathed about 25 patients before I went to Jane's room.

Ah, Jane.

Jane weighed more than 700 pounds, and she was immobile due to her weight and the conditions she developed because of her size and lifestyle. She was particularly difficult to work with, and I say that in the nicest way possible. The truth is, working with Jane was anything but pleasant. It was a freaking nightmare. It was hell. Everyone dreaded it.

Jane was abusive—verbally and physically—to staff, and so much that the facility threatened to kick her out several times. Her family, though, ponied up more and more money each time, and money talks. Jane knew her behavior was swept under the rug, so she became progressively worse and was allowed to do anything she wanted. The facility director told us to 'just take it' from Jane and 'never tell her no.' Every few months, a few nurses would quit or threaten a lawsuit, and then the director would go back to Jane's family. It was a vicious, tired cycle.

We were all Jane's personal servants. I was warned about her on my first day, and by the end of the day, Jane had me fetching her Cheetos, dozens of sodas, leaving post to buy her Taco Bell and Captain D's, and helping her install apps on the laptop that she'd received from her family. A year later, nothing had really changed, except I made it a point to never pass her room unless she already a servant for the day.

I bathed Jane at her bedside that day. It took about thirty minutes to clean under all her folds, and that was not counting the 'roll break,' which is when we utilized the services of four nurses and a lifting belt to move Jane, so we could wash her backside.

When it was time to dry and dress Jane, she demanded baby powder. Well, baby powder had just been banned at our facility due to health concerns (inhaling talc was the highest concern, but it was noted that baby powder may break down and/or irritate skin over time, with consistent usage). Still, Jane demanded baby powder. I politely informed her a second time that the facility banned baby powder, and her response to that was to bite me. I screamed, another aide entered the room, and I used a rag to clean the blood from my wound.

I was at my wit's end, until the fellow aide informed me there were cans of aerosol baby powder in our supply room. He said this in front of Jane, so she ordered me out of the room to fetch some. She told me not to come back until I had baby powder and a cup of rice pudding from the cafeteria. Her idea of a cup of rice pudding was an actual 32-ounce Styrofoam cup filled with the pudding. She drank it through a plastic smoothie straw.

I was livid, I'll admit that. I was sick and tired of being bossed around by this monster. I sure wasn't getting paid enough to put up with that kind of abuse. The stress that came with working with Jane left me feeling depressed and angry all the time. When I went home at night, all I wanted to do was drink to forget how she'd hit me and called me names. I couldn't stand getting up when my alarm went off in the mornings, because all I could think about was how bad it'd be with Jane that day. I loved every other patient there, and I loved my job. It was Jane. Her poor behavior overshadowed the positivity in my career.

I went to the supply room and saw a bunch of aerosol cans on the third shelf, right where my coworker said they'd be. I wasn't in the room more than ten seconds. Then, I went to the cafeteria, grabbed a cup, and stood in a long line until I could have the cafeteria worker fill it with pudding.

"This is her second one today," the worker told me, shaking her head.

I frowned because, right at that moment, I actually felt bad for Jane.

That didn't last long, I can tell you that.

When I went in the room, Jane cursed at me and demanded that I walk faster to deliver her pudding-cup. She ordered me to find her smoothie straw. She threw a book at me because her soap opera had been replaced by breaking news. Oh, she was getting on my last nerve.

Jane spread her legs and told me to put baby powder on her buttocks, thighs, and then lift her rolls and powder those areas too.

When I moved near the end of the bed and moved in to powder Jane, she said, "This is what I think of you."

She then passed gas.

I furiously shook the can of baby powder, moved in close, and just really put my finger down hard to spray as much as I possibly could and get it done as fast as I could.

I was so worked up and moving so fast that it honestly took me a minute to realize I smelled pine trees.

"It stings!" Jane yelled. "You stupid bitch, what did you do to me?"

I panicked and looked at the can.

It wasn't baby powder. I had grabbed a can of air freshener.

I hurried to wash the chemicals from Jane's genitals and thighs, but I couldn't even do that because she kicked me in the face. She kicked me so hard that she broke my nose and I had to go to an emergency dentist because one of my teeth came loose. There was nothing they could do, so that tooth fell out and I had to get an implant. My job didn't carry insurance, so I had to pay for that out of pocket. With the dental bills and ER co-pay, I paid almost $7,000 after Jane kicked me. I had to max out a credit card and borrow money from my mom.

Jane reported me to the facility director, and because I 'caused the patient distress and potentially bodily harm,' I was terminated. I am not saying that I was innocent because I should have been more careful when grabbing the can from the supply room, but what I did was not intentional. Even though I hated working with Jane, I would have never compromised her safety. I take my job seriously.

It took me almost a month to find another job because I had to list that employment on my applications, and it never looks good when you've been terminated. Finally, I was hired by another long-term facility, and I've been here four years.

I honestly don't know what happened to Jane, and I don't care. Maybe she had reasons for behaving that way, but I won't allow anyone to make excuses for treating others so badly. I don't feel sorry for her at all. I do feel sorry for all the other aides and nurses she abused.

--Initials and location withheld at request

<u>Cross-Training</u>

Where I work, RNs and techs began cross-training for ED registration about a year ago. Our admin thought this cross-training would allow for faster recognition of life-saving intervention, as registration clerks may not always be capable of identifying emergency distresses, such as labored breathing or similar symptoms. Admin also thought it would be a good idea to help nurses experience how the registration department felt, noting several registration clerks had recently quit, citing RNs' attitudes. None of us thought that was our problem. I don't know why you guys think you deserve more than minimum wage to answer a damn phone, and why do you think we should have to be nice to you? Just do what we tell you and shut up.

Let me tell you this: I know you worked in registration, and I know plenty others do it to, but I always thought that's a job for you guys, not us. Look, it's a simple fact: when you pull nurses from the floor and tell them to file paperwork all night, it's a waste of resources. I certainly didn't go to school to sit on my butt and eat chips while browsing the internet all night like the normal registration girls up front. So, none of us were happy about the cross-training, especially because on days we were scheduled for registration duty, our hourly pay decreased as a 'scaling income to workload' policy.

One night I was on registration duty, and I was already frustrated because I was losing about five-dollars an hour. It had been busy, too, and I was frustrated that I was losing money, but essentially was still up to my neck in work. It made zero-effing-sense, and it wasn't fair.

I have to admit, I am also used to being in charge or being able to have the final word in an argument with a patient. As an RN, if I tell you no, that doesn't mean you can go talk to someone else and have that cup of water. It means you get no water. As a clerk, however, since I wasn't the RN for the patient, I could *suggest* they couldn't have water prior to being seen, but I couldn't flat out tell them no.

Patients were challenging everything I said. I even had patients cursing and spitting at me because I told them to wait in the waiting room. Your three-day-old does not have COPD, okay? She probably has a cold because you decided to take her to the mall and pass her around to total germ-ridden strangers right after you pushed her out your vagina. 98.9 is not a fever, she's not crying, and there are simply no indications to suggest that I flag you as a priority patient. Go—sit—down and stop telling me that you have to be seen *right now.*

It had been about four hours, and being an RN had nothing to do with the shift so far. It was pointless. I could understand why registration clerks came back to see us so often, though, because these patients were so used to saying they were filing complaints and registration clerks were under strict customer service regulations, that I started to understand it all. I didn't have to go back to check symptoms with nurses or ask if a patient with an ankle injury could have an ice pack because I already knew those answers.

I started thinking back on all the times I'd called various registration girls idiots—to their faces or behind their backs—and I have to say, I started regretting my behavior. As the shift continued, I could understand why these clerks were often on the verge of tears or looked exhausted. I think about every other patient cursed and yelled at me that night. It felt like I was telling someone to wait their turn about every five minutes, and people didn't seem to understand that just one person can't be taking an admit call *and* talk to a patient standing at the desk with his finger caught in a mouse trap. I was just one person with two arms, okay? And I was being paid a shitty wage to sit there and tolerate that kind of behavior and present nothing but a sweet smile back.

I went to my boss and informed her that I would *not* be returning to the registration position, and I told her she could fire me if she wanted to. I told her that maybe we should give the registration clerks a raise and hire a second clerk, just to help with the workload up there. My boss didn't fire me. She marked my name off a list, and she said that was the point of cross-training. (And I was never in danger of losing that five-dollars an hour, anyway—we were told that to make us angry, but it showed up on our checks as a bonus.) Registration would still be paid less than nurses, but the training was to show that just because they were paid less and did not have professional medical training, did not mean they did not have hard jobs.

The hospital continues with mandatory cross-training in our department, and I can tell the difference. Sure, there are some RNs who still treat registration poorly and look down on registration, but I am no longer one of those people. It took me one night to realize how hard those clerks work and what they have to deal with. It was like being in retail, where the customer is always right, even when they're assaulting you, and dealing with people who are whining about a non-existent fever while there are people bleeding to death in the back. It was hell, and I never want to do that job again.

--J.M.
California

Unfaithful

One time, this lady and her man walked inside. I remember the night quite well because it had been storming pretty badly, so we were slow. I called security as the two stood in the lobby and shouted at one another. They didn't even care that I was sitting there, or that there were people in the waiting room.

Security told the two to either register or leave, so the man tried to leave, and this started another round between the two. A nurse came to the front to find out what was wrong, and I explained that I wasn't sure yet, but the couple had been fighting from the get-go.

Finally, after the woman was finished arguing with security about how she'd been fighting with her man, both came to the intake desk. I sat up straight and treated them as if I hadn't watched them fight for 10 minutes. I felt awkward.

"Who's the patient tonight?" I asked.

The woman pointed to the man and said, "My boyfriend needs to see a doctor. And I'm going with him, so don't even tell me I can't."

The nurse made a 'humph' noise that was barely audible and I just said, "Uh, okay. What's going on tonight?"

The woman folded her arms over her chest and said bitterly, "Well, tell them, John. What seems to be the problem?"

"She's crazy," he said to me. "I think she needs to see a mental doctor."

"I am not crazy!" the woman shrieked.

Security took a step forward, but it was the nurse who spoke up and said, "Okay, let's knock off the fighting. I'm sick of it already, and since I'm the triage nurse, I can and will separate you two if you can't get along."

The man snickered, which set the woman off again, and off to the races they went.

Security stepped in again, and the woman screamed at me, "He'd screw you, you know. But it's not a compliment; he'll screw anything that moves."

I remember a story you told, one where a patient turned on you out of the blue, and I felt much the same way. I was thinking, 'Gee whiz, what did I do to you, lady?'

"I have never cheated on you!" the man shouted.

"Then why does your dick smell that way?" yelled the girlfriend.

Whaaaaaaa?

I swear, security, the nurse, and I were all looking at each other like we were watching a live taping of *Jerry Springer*.

"I didn't cheat on you, okay?" the man screamed. "I don't know what you think my dick smells like. I don't know what it usually smells like, but I didn't do anything different with it."

"You were sleeping with that slut from work," the girlfriend accused.

"Ms. Doe? Why do you keep saying that?"

"Because you always talk about her and send her texts! I know you're sleeping with her."

"She's sixty-four," the man yelled. "She's about to retire and it's my job to answer her questions. It's not just her; I help anyone who needs help. That's my job!"

"Then who have you been sleeping with? Your dick wouldn't smell like another [vagina] if you weren't sticking it in one."

The man grabbed his face with his hand and groaned. "I told you already, I am not cheating on you."

Security interrupted the couple again, and the woman yelled at me, "Well, why aren't you getting us back to a doctor?"

I stammered, "I…I don't know what you want me to do right now. I don't know what to put as your symptoms."

The woman growled and said, "I want a doctor to look at his dick and test it. I want to know if there's another woman's [vagina] on his dick."

"Uhhh," I said.

I looked back to the nurse with this expression that pleaded, 'help me.'

"Ma'am," the nurse stated, "we don't test for anything like that. This seems like a domestic dispute, not a medical emergency."

"I know the doctor can do the test," the woman snapped. "Don't stand there and tell me lies."

"Ma'am," the nurse repeated, "there is nothing we can do. We can run STD checks, but for something like that, I would recommend visiting your PCP."

The woman shook her head and said, "Uh-uh. We're not going anywhere until this is settled."

"Baby," the man whined, "let's just go home. I'll go to the doctor with you in the morning."

"Don't you 'baby' me," the woman replied. "And we're not leaving. You're going to see a doctor, and he's going to tell us for sure if you've been hoeing around."

The nurse skipped the triage process and took the couple straight to the back. Security had to stand outside the room and I heard them yelling off and on.

I guess the man's STD tests came back negative, but like they were already informed, there were no tests to determine if the man had cheated on his girlfriend. As they were leaving, it was clear that she still believed he'd been cheating on her, although he was adamant that he never cheated.

--H.E.
Louisiana

Paging, Doctor Uncaring

I do not want to disclose too much of my patient's condition, but I can tell you that he was transferred from another facility to our ICU. His admission was approved by our on-call physician over a direct admit call. During a direct admit call, a physician from each facility will discuss the patient's condition. In this case, the patient was doing well, but still needed to be transferred to our facility as a safety precaution, as our facility is more advanced than the patient's original admitting facility.

Our patient was admitted as to an ICU Level I bed. This means the patient required little staff support and was receiving oxygen via nasal cannula. His vitals were stable upon arrival. He seemed alert and aware of his surroundings, but he requested 'something to knock [him] out.' We checked his orders and he was receiving a drip at his previous facility.

Our doctor had already reviewed the medication list and approved that he could have the drip at our hospital. I administered the drip per order and the patient fell asleep.

Please keep in mind that the accepting physician from our facility was not present on the floor. He had taken the direct admit call from home.

Within an hour of the patient's admission to our floor, he coded.

Of course, we called the code and were required to page Dr. Smith. After two minutes, Dr. Smith never returned my page. Naturally, I suspected switchboard made an error or that the doctor did not receive the page for whatever reason. I had him paged again. He still did not respond.

With the help of ancillary departments, the patient was stabilized, and we called Registration to change the patient's bed status from Level I to Level II, meaning he now required more care and more staff monitoring.

Soon after, the patient coded again.

Again, I paged Dr. Smith.

No reply.

I paged him again.

No reply.

Once we stabilized the patient, I personally used our web-paging application to page Dr. Smith. That way, I would know that I typed in the correct number, sent the correct message, and I would have peace of mind.

No reply.

I cannot tell you how frustrated I was at this point. Even other RNs were complaining that they'd also paged Dr. Smith, and he was not replying. Our House Super commented that she could not reach him.

I took matters into my own hands and I asked switchboard to connect me to Dr. Smith's personal home number. She refused, citing that Dr. Smith's preferred method of contact while he was on-call was his pager, and that she could not connect calls to him in any other fashion.

Twenty dollars from my purse helped her 'accidentally' click on his home phone number. (That money was supposed to be used to buy myself Girl Scout cookies, so I'm still really pissed about that. It was the last day to buy them, so I missed out and had to pay $3 more per box to get them from another nurse the following week.)

The phone rang three times, before Dr. Smith abrasively answered, "Hello?"

"Dr. Smith?" I asked. "Is your pager broken?"

I could hear him chewing food and there were loud voices and noises in the background.

"No," he said.

"The patient we just accepted from that direct admit has coded twice."

"Okay."

OKAY? OKAY? That's all you're going to say about this? Oh, I was livid!

"I had you paged multiple times. I even sent a web-page through myself."

"I saw," he said, sounding rather distracted.

"Ooh," he exclaimed. "Got that one right in the face."

"Excuse me?" I asked.

"Look, sweetie," he said to me, "I'm watching a movie right now."

"But, your patient—," I started to say.

"What did I just say? I said, I'm watching a movie right now. Look, sweetie, I have to go."

Dr. Smith then hung up on me.

When I asked switchboard to reconnect me, she did (at no extra cost). Dr. Smith's line rang busy and he did not reply to another page.

I was marching straight to find the House Super, when I passed a group of RNs griping about being unable to reach Dr. Smith to clarify orders. Some of their patients were in pain and needed meds that only Dr. Smith could approve or alter.

"He's watching a movie, don't you know?" I said bitterly.

"Huh?" one of the RNs asked me.

I explained the short conversation I'd just had with Dr. Smith, and the other RNs were also livid.

"Well," one said, "I'm paging him. I suggest you do the same."

"It won't work," I said with a huff. "He's ignoring the pages."

The RN shrugged and said, "It doesn't mean that I can't flood his pager."

This group of five RNs (six, if you count me) used switchboard and our web-paging application to page Dr. Smith more than *two hundred* times in a matter of minutes. They'd sent so many pages through the online system that they crashed it and I.T. had to do a soft reset of that system. I don't think it caused major problems, but it did cause a minor upset, just because so many people relied on it in the facility. Once they found out what happened, they supported our 'cause' and found it humorous.

I still notified the House Super. She was so mad that I think she was red in the face for the rest of her shift.

Dr. Smith came walking in like nothing had happened about an hour after all the pages. One RN walked out on her shift (she was cited but was encouraged and allowed to return at a later date), and the other RNs basically ganged up on Dr. Smith in the hallway. He was incredibly sexist and dismissive of our arguments. Once confronted by the Super, Dr. Smith relinquished his patients' care to another physician, who'd been called at home for a facility emergency and graciously agreed to take control of Dr. Smith's patients.

Dr. Smith was terminated, following a formal hearing. He tried to say that nobody had paged him, but switchboard documents all pages and stat calls to physicians. Also, H.R. used those 200-something pages as proof that staff, indeed, did attempt to contact Dr. Smith. I had to give a statement and recall the phone call to multiple people as part of the investigation.

--D.H.

Location withheld at request

That's Nuts

At my hospital, we only have one intake clerk on shift at any given time. Our hospital is not particularly small but our patients, thank the Lord, only seem to come to the ER when they *really* need to. Every now and then, we will get moms who bring in kids for stupid stuff, like occasionally we'll get a kid in for head lice or because the kid has a 'rash' on their face, which turns out to be a stain from a popsicle. For the most part, though, we only see true emergencies, and we usually only see about 10 patients per shift. On a busy shift, we'll maybe see about 15, so it can be hectic at times, but it's usually manageable. It helps that our hospital allows us to eat on shift (at our desk), and staff supports each other.

Well, one day, this car pulled up in front of the ER. I couldn't see the driver. Minutes later, this large (by weight and height) man got out of the car. He looked like he could've been a football player in his younger days, just because he was so tall. I figured he'd always been a bigger man by weight, but now he must have weighed 400-pounds, at least. I could tell he was in bad shape before he even reached the door, so I called for help.

The man managed to enter the lobby and leaned against the wall. He was gasping for air, his skin appeared dark yellow and clammy, and he could only pat at his chest and say, "I need help."

Two nurses put the man in a wheelchair and took him straight back. I guess tests determined that he was having serious heart problems. (I'm sorry, I am not a nurse and don't know anything about this stuff. I can only tell you what others told me and what I witnessed.)

The unit clerk called up to me and told me to hurry to the patient's room and get him registered.

The patient handed me his wallet and said there were papers inside that detailed his contact and insurance information.

While I was in the room, the doctor asked, "How long have you had kidney failure?"

The patient replied, "Kidney failure? My kidneys are dying?"

I rushed to my desk and registered the patient.

The long story short here is that the patient was in severe condition. He apparently told the doctor that his wife passed away the year before, so he turned to food as a coping mechanism. His favorite comfort food was peanut butter, so he would eat between two and three 'family jars' per day!

I guess he had high phosphorus levels and had calcium deposits in his heart and blood vessels.

This patient was in our ER for a few hours, before he was life-lined to another hospital a few hours away—something that we rarely encounter at this hospital.

Now, I don't know if the excessive consumption of peanut butter caused this, but I heard the doctor talking about how the patient had untreated and undiagnosed diabetes, kidney failure, and CHF. Those were the big conditions I remember, but I know he had several more issues. The patient apparently had not visited a doctor in more than 20 years.

I've never seen or heard of anything like this, so I thought it would be worth sharing with you and your other readers. If anything, I guess it can be used to remind people that checkups are important, and that moderation is key when consuming any food.

--Initials withheld at request

Wyoming

Round and Round We Go

This was a first in my EMS career. It happened a while back, but I still have no words.

We responded to a complaint of a pedestrian struck by a motor vehicle at an abandoned park in a rural community. The town has a population of roughly 300 people, and the town is located approximately 30 minutes from the nearest Band-Aid station. The park is located in an odd place. See, the park is about five minutes away from the town center, and it's surrounded by fields. It makes no sense to me that someone would ever build a park there, but I guess some hundred years ago, the town's population lived nearer to the park.

Anyway, we sped to the park, cutting a 35-minute trip (we always check our gear before going on a run) down to about a 20-minute trip. Yeah, we were booking it.

When we pulled up to the park—which was basically a merry-go-round, two swings on a rusty frame, and an old metal slide with holes in it from erosion—my mind instantly went, 'What in the hell is this?'

The first thing I noticed was a dirt bike on the ground, with a thick metal chain running from an anchor at the end of the bike, to one of the handles on the merry-go-round. The bike was still running, kicking up dust.

Right next to the bike, to the eastern side of the merry-go-round, there was a male, in his mid-to-late-20s, kneeling over a female. The female was squealing like a pig.

To the northern side of the merry-go-round, there were two females, also in their 20s, sitting on the ground, crying, and holding their legs.

To the western side of the merry-go-round, there was what appeared to be an unconscious male.

On the merry-go-round itself was one female, sitting with her head dipped between her legs. There was a pool of vomit at her feet.

Please, can someone explain how I end up dispatched to all of these batshit crazy runs?

I did and didn't want to know what happened, but I knew I was about to hear it, anyway.

Okay, so these idiots decided that since they couldn't get drunk on a Sunday (county law that you can't buy alcohol), they were going to go to the park to try someone's 'good idea.'

Apparently, one male and one female were going to stand on the merry-go-round, while a male on the dirt bike used the chain to rotate the merry-go-round as fast as it would go. There were three female bystanders. Two bystanders' legs were apparently struck when they moved in the way, and the third bystander was struck by the dirt bike. The male merry-go-round rider was thrown from the equipment, while the female rider remained on the equipment, only suffering from motion sickness and dizziness.

Of the group, only two required what we would consider 'true emergencies.' The female who was struck by the dirt bike required medical attention (she sustained

161

internal bleeding), and the male thrown from the ride sustained head and neck injuries. The bystanders with the leg injuries appeared to have heavy bruising to their calves, the female rider stopped vomiting and went right for a 20-ounce of Mountain Dew and smoked two cigarettes, and the dirt bike operator was in perfect physical condition.

All six patients requested medical transport. The girls with the bruising said they wanted x-rays, the barfing girl said she wanted an ultrasound to check on the condition of her ten-week-old fetus (WTF?!), and the dirt bike operator said he needed 'some oxys or something' because he was 'depressed' over slamming his bike into his friend's girlfriend.

We had to call for backup because we'd only been expecting to transport one patient.

Of the six, the two I told you about (the girl who'd been struck by the bike and the guy who'd been thrown off the equipment) were admitted to the ER at our Band-Aid station, and then they were transported by helicopter to a trauma center four hours away.

I hope I never see anything else like this for the remainder of my career. I mean, the injuries weren't too bad to witness, but if I have to encounter another group of people so dumb, I might go to jail for beating them all.

--X.K.
Illinois

Mr. Fix-It?

Way back in the day, before cell phones and Google, we had to do things the 'old fashioned' way. If we needed a mechanic, we went on down to Dave's garage, or we opened the Yellow Pages and found someone who could work on our cars. The problem with this method in the good ol' days is that in small towns, not everyone got along all the time.

My neighbor, John, had a tree he needed to down—and quick—or it was going to come down in a real bad way during a summer storm. Well, John had a bone to pick with Jim, who was our local tree trimmer. John absolutely refused to give Jim any business. John was positive he could down the tree himself, saying (while he was six beers in and about to finish his seventh), "Come on, it can't be that hard."

My wife and I told John not to cut the tree himself. His wife told him not to cut the tree himself. Other neighbors told him not to cut the tree himself.

So, naturally, John cut the tree himself.

John thought it would be a fantastic idea to get up at the crack of dawn and use a chainsaw at the base of this 33-foot Oak.

I guess my wife and I slept through the racket, for the most part. But, I do remember my wife shaking me awake and asking, "What's that sound?"

Not even thirty seconds later, as my wife and I were lying in the dark, a tree tore through our roof.

Luckily, my wife and I were uninjured, but John's wife was not so lucky. In a way, I suppose she *was* lucky. The tree sliced both our homes in half, and I mean that quite literally. The tree was lying in the middle of our demolished homes. It looked like a tornado had come through. John's wife was hit by a limb from the falling tree, and she broke her arm. She had to get a few dozen stitches to her face, too, from getting hit with branches and debris.

John was arrested at almost 06:00 for his public intoxication and his dangerous tree-downing. Thankfully, John's insurance took care of the cost of both homes, but it was heated in our neighborhood for a good few years after the incident.

To top off the absurdity of my story, let me add that John and Jim worked out their differences about a *week* after this happened, so if he would have just waited a lousy seven days, maybe I wouldn't have had to go through that.

John and I are still on speaking terms (we weren't for a very long time), but I still bring up the incident any chance I can get.

Last beer in the cooler at the cookout? "Hey, remember when you cut down that tree and destroyed my house?"

--A.J. Y.
Kentucky

Friendly Reminder from an LEO:

If you're going to bail your friend out of jail, it's best *not* to pay us in fake bills or write us a stolen check.

--N.C.
Utah

Beautiful Day in the Neighborhood

I moved to this town because I was offered a position on OB, so it only made sense to relocate, rather than commute an hour each way. That way, I wouldn't have to call in due to poor weather conditions, and I wouldn't have to struggle with time zones and my schedule.

When I first moved here four years ago, this neighborhood appeared somewhat rundown, but quiet. During the summer, I'd occasionally see a druggie staggering down the road or a drunk falling off the sidewalk at night. Every now and then, a few neighbors would have one too many and scuffle. For the most part, however, it was safe and quiet.

That all changed last summer. Drugs have always been present in this town, but last summer, the drug scene exploded. Even 'high class' neighborhoods experienced higher levels of vandalism and 911 calls for drunk and high suspects. My neighborhood went downhill fast. During the warmer months, it wasn't unusual to see cops on the block several times per night. Breaking and entering became more common. Someone busted out my driver's side window, just to steal an expired coupon from McDonald's. I started leaving my doors unlocked because I wiped out my savings to pay the insurance deductible, and I couldn't afford another incident. That's why I didn't move, too; I may be a nurse, but I have bills like everyone else. I just bought the house, too. There was no way I could sell and get the money I paid.

One night, I left work a little after midnight. When I pulled in my driveway, I noticed my living room light was on. I didn't remember leaving it on. I knew I left the kitchen light on, because my coworkers said to try to leave at least one light on when I left the house to give the illusion that someone is home. I started thinking that maybe I did leave the light on. It had been a long shift and I was exhausted, so I just didn't think much of it as I got out of my car.

My front door was still locked, so that was a good sign. I thought so, anyway.

When I got inside, I was floored. Someone had broken my bedroom window, entered my house, and robbed me. They took my TV and all my electronics, my washer and dryer, my furniture (including my bed—they left my mattress and bedding), went through my closet, took jewelry that my deceased grandmother had given me, a new cooking set, and they even took my phone charger.

When I called the police, they said they couldn't really do much. They told me to watch pawn shops and the yard sale groups on Facebook.

My insurance took care of the financial loss (again), but they couldn't cover sentimental value, or the stress involved in the incident.

As soon as the insurance check came in, I bought a dog before I bought anything else. I went to a breeder recommended by a coworker and found a trained German Shepherd. She didn't fully ease my mind but having her helped.

Fast forward to last week.

The neighborhood has gotten even worse since the break in. Now, we have this man who walks around and screams at people. He appears to be on drugs when I see him. Officers have been called, but apparently, they have no reason to arrest him. They just talk to him and send him back to terrorize the rest of us.

Last week, I was hanging out with my neighbors on my first night off in fifteen days (we are severely short-staffed right now, so I am scheduled 15-18 shifts on, with one off in between until we are back to full staff). We were all drinking, although not heavily, and we had a fire going in the pit.

Well, as we were enjoying ourselves, the man who screams at people did just that. He walked onto the neighbors' property and began threatening the neighbor, right there in front of the man's pregnant wife, child, and other neighbors. We diffused the situation and the 'crazy' man went on his way.

We didn't think much of this incident because it's become so common to experience this.

About two hours later, the crazy man returned, and his behavior was much more erratic. He was threatening all of us, but this time seemed more focused on the neighbor's wife and child. When he screamed at the child that he was going to come back at night and kill her, the situation went from bad to worse. The neighbor, a veteran, approached the crazy man, and we thought it was going to be a quick knockout.

Instead, the crazy man grabbed from a pile of debris at the side of the yard, and he began throwing bricks at us. The neighbor still attempted to stop this man's behavior.

Before we knew it, the crazy man whipped out a machete-type knife from his waistband. The blade on this knife must have been at least seven-inches long. He sliced at the neighbor's abdomen and then began attempting to stab the neighbor.

The neighbor jumped back, and the crazy man retreated to an aluminum storage shack in a nearby yard.

At first, we thought it had been a tense situation with no injuries.

"Can you believe that guy?" the neighbor exclaimed, as he turned to us.

His toddler began sobbing and saying, "Daddy hurt."

My neighbor's tee shirt was saturated with blood, and there was blood just pouring to the ground.

He lifted his shirt to show a deep laceration that was approximately ten-inches in length. Then, in true soldier fashion, he said as if it were no big deal, "Huh, look at that."

Another neighbor removed his shirt and I used it to apply pressure to my other neighbor's wound.

Within two minutes of this altercation, ten police cars arrived, and I think I counted fifteen officers from the Sheriff's Department, our local PD, and the State Police. (We still don't know who called the cops because it wasn't any of us.) Two ambulances arrived shortly after, along with one fire truck.

Officers took statements from all six of us and went to the shed to speak to the suspect. I guess he'd fled while we were focused on the neighbor's wound, so it was a great feeling to know that there was a crazy man running around town with a machete and he obviously was prepared to use the weapon.

At my neighbors' request, I drove the wife and child to the ER, while the injured husband was transported via ambulance. I watched their child while the husband received 22 sutures to his wound.

When he and his wife emerged from the ER, I asked how it went. He shrugged and said, "I was shot in the head when I was overseas, so this is nothing."

Against the ER doctor's and my advice, the neighbor went home and decided to continue drinking around the fire pit. Things calmed down, and his wife put their toddler to bed and came back outside.

We were having a great time, joking, and talking. We even threw some more food over the fire and were all enjoying ourselves. I leashed my dog and brought her over to sit with us.

As we were joking around, my dog stood at attention. I looked up and gasped. The crazy man had walked onto the property again and was just standing there, watching us.

My neighbor told the man to leave, and his wife started to dial 911 on her cell phone. When the crazy man realized she was calling for help, he rushed at her.

My dog, without a command to do so, ran at full speed and got to the pregnant woman before her husband did. She stood between the woman and the crazy man, and she was prepared to bite. When the man attempted to hit the pregnant neighbor, my dog did bite. She held until the woman was able to move to a safe distance and until the crazy man stopped struggling, even though he punched my dog several times and poked her in the eyes in an attempt to make her let go.

Just like earlier, officers swarmed the neighborhood and transported the crazy man to the hospital for treatment. He received a few sutures for a clean bite, and then he was transported to jail.

Unfortunately, he was back on the streets after two nights in jail. I guess he's supposed to appear in court in a few weeks. It is disheartening and scary to see how our justice system operates. We are hoping he will be picked up again before his court date, and that this next time he will be held longer.

I sustained two broken fingers from getting caught in the leash when my dog rushed to protect the neighbor. Some people were saying it wasn't 'right' for a trained dog to react that way, but I'm not worried at all because she did what I would expect a dog to do in that situation, and she saved the neighbor from being assaulted. Who knows if he would've tried to stab her before her husband could intervene?

My coworkers all said they felt sorry for me. Most of them read about the incident on Facebook, and there was an article in the local paper about what happened.

So much for that being a relaxing day off.

--Initials and location withheld at request

Animal Farm

Every year, residents come together to host a fundraiser for a random illness at our SNF. Last year, we had a bake sale, cake walk, and silent auction to raise money for Lymphoma. This year, we had a bake sale, some of our residents thought it would be fun to play live music, and we held a small rummage sale with items donated by residents, their families, and the community.

Usually, these events are busy and fun. The community comes together and there are usually local vendors with booths, also selling items and/or food to contribute to the fundraiser.

One year, a petting zoo contacted us and offered its services for a fundraiser for preemie babies. We thought this would be a fantastic idea. Our residents were not allowed to have pets at our facility, and we had a few newcomers who'd surrendered their animals to move in with us. We thought a petting zoo would boost morale with our residents and be a lot of fun for kids, since our fundraisers are usually more geared toward adults.

Everything seemed to be going fine. Our residents were manning their baked goods stations, mingling with the community, and some were enjoying face painting or watching the amateur magician. The turnout was great. We must have had more than 200 people there that day, not including our residents and staff.

About an hour before calling it a day, one of the petting zoo employees was frantically approaching people, asking if anyone had seen a gray pygmy goat.

Hmm, what an odd question!

Soon, the petting zoo owner was questioning the public, explaining that they were missing a kid (goat, that is) that was estimated to be about 30 pounds. The owner and his staff thought the goat somehow managed to escape. He and his staff spread out to search the facility grounds and surrounding area.

I went inside to check on some of the residents who'd tired out or simply refused to join in on the event.

For the most part, the residents were doing fine. Some were rather grumpy and didn't even want to talk to me, but others let me know they were doing okay and went back to needlepoint or watching television.

As I approached the end of the hall, I heard an odd noise and couldn't quite figure out what I had heard, exactly.

I went to Mr. Smith's room. Mr. Smith was 82-years-old at the time, and he was the sweetest resident. He never caused us an ounce of grief, and he helped a great deal of newcomers adapt to living with us.

For the first time in years, Mr. Smith's door was closed. Red flag.

When I opened the door, Mr. Smith was sitting on the edge of his bed, with the missing goat on his lap. The goat was wearing an oversized tee shirt. Mr. Smith was feeding the goat sunflower seeds out of the palm of his hand, and they were both watching the nightly news.

"Mr. Smith!" I exclaimed.

This man suddenly became someone I did not know. He began shouting, demanding that

I leave immediately. He held the goat tightly to his chest and screamed that I could not take the goat. Mr. Smith said he was petting the goat and decided that 'Billy' would be happier living in Mr. Smith's room, rather than live in a petting zoo.

After minutes of attempting to convince Mr. Smith to hand Billy over to me, he became violent. He placed the goat on his bed and threw a chair at me. I had no choice but to find my supervisor and notify the petting zoo owner.

The supervisor, two orderlies, the petting zoo owner, and I all attempted to convince Mr. Smith to surrender the goat. He continued throwing furniture and belongings at us. His behavior was so violent that nobody could enter his room. We had to negotiate with Mr. Smith at his door. It was a hostage situation at this point, in a way. Mr. Smith never threatened to hurt Billy, but he threatened several times to hurt himself. He broke a vase and warned us to stay away, or he'd use a piece of ceramic to cut his throat. We didn't know what to do.

My supervisor called the police and EMS because of the nature of Mr. Smith's threats. Residents had gathered in the halls. It was a hectic scene.

Before the police arrived, one of our residents came to Mr. Smith's door and miraculously convinced him that Billy was better off in the petting zoo. She reminded Mr. Smith that the goat required food and medical care that we could not provide. Mr. Smith reluctantly and tearfully returned Billy to the petting zoo owner.

Thankfully, the owner did not wish to press charges. Unfortunately, due to the nature of the incident, Mr. Smith's family demanded that he be taken to the hospital for a mental health evaluation. Because he had threatened suicide, he was held for mandatory observation. After it was determined that Mr. Smith was of sound mind and suffered from what he called 'temporary passionate insanity,' he was returned to our center.

Mr. Smith apologized to all of us and personally apologized for throwing a chair at me. He told me he missed having a pet and that he was lonely because his family never came around anymore.

It took a while, but we now have two facility cats that our residents care for. Mr. Smith is still around and is active in caring for the cats.

--D.O.
Oklahoma

Under Attack

In one of your books, you included tips from EMTs. One of the tips said to crate pets, if possible, before EMS arrived. I cannot stress enough how important that advice is!

Years ago, my partner and I were dispatched to a residence. The caller complained of chest pain and dizziness. She remained on the line but became unresponsive to the operator while we were en route.

When we arrived on scene and approached the house, we listened for any signs of dogs in the residence. We didn't hear anything, so we went inside.

An older woman was lying on the kitchen floor. She was not breathing and had no pulse.

We attempted to revive the patient by performing chest compressions.

While we were doing this, there was a loud crash from the back part of the house.

I didn't even have time to react when I saw two large mixed-breed dogs running at me.

I don't know if the dogs thought we had hurt their owner, or if they were just territorial, but they attacked me.

My partner attempted to pull the dogs off me, and I managed to yank my arm away from one. When I jerked away, a chunk of my arm went with the dog. It flung my flesh from its mouth before attacking me again.

Not knowing what else to do, my partner hit the dogs with a heavy statue-thing that was holding the kitchen door open. They still wouldn't stop attacking me. My partner dispatched for animal control and officers. Dispatch suggested tossing a blanket over the dogs, which I guess would possibly disorient them. That did not work, so dispatch then suggested splashing the dogs with cold water. That helped.

I passed out. I lost more than two pints of blood at the scene and went into shock.

Unfortunately, the homeowner was declared dead and her dogs (who'd knocked down a baby gate to get out of her bedroom) were put down. I understand that not everyone thinks that was the best decision, but these dogs mauled me. I have undergone more than a dozen surgeries to my arms and face, and I received more than 175 stitches. I still have nerve damage to my arms and fingers. In fact, I cannot feel in my fingertips on two fingers, and one of my fingers was amputated. If it had not been for my partner, I think the dogs would have killed me.

From that moment on, I have been afraid of dogs. I had to give my own dog to a family member because I could not even look at him without having a panic attack. My former employer paid for therapy, and now I can encounter dogs with a slightly better reaction than crying and hyperventilating, but I do not think I will ever be able to come within 20 feet of a dog ever again.

--E.W.
California

I am an EMT but transport so many B.S. calls that I now identify as a taxi driver.

I wish I could charge a cash fare to all these people who call us for rides to the hospital, just so they can LBT and go to the fast food places across the street.

--M.U.
New Jersey

Oops

It was 03:00, and I was standing in front of the coffee machine in the hallway, kind of zoning out as it was preparing my two-dollar 'cappuccino.' I work on ICU and can only say it had been a long shift.

As I was waiting on my drink, this guy came from the ER waiting room and stood next to me, in front of the food vending machine. I kind of glanced at him, but I didn't want to make eye contact or give him a reason to think I wanted to talk. Sometimes, when I buy coffee from that machine, families from the ER waiting room think I'm an ER nurse, so they bombard me with questions or come out of nowhere with anger and accusations. I wasn't in the mood that night. I just wanted to get my crappy, overpriced coffee, then go find an empty bathroom where I could sit on the floor and daydream about winning the lottery and buying a mansion in France.

The protective cover on the coffee machine opened and I took my coffee, just as the man next to me started digging in his pocket (for change, I assume).

The next thing I knew, a gunshot scared the crap out of me. I threw my steaming cup of coffee in the air. It splattered all over me, and I instantly knew my burns would require medical attention.

At first, I didn't know what was going on. I could hear people screaming from down the hall. The ER clerks must have hit the panic alarm, because the metal covering came down over their glass window, and an automated message over the speakers announced a Code Silver, which is a situation in which a weapon is involved.

I looked over and saw the man rolling around on the ground. He was bleeding from a GSW to his upper thigh. The amount of blood he was losing was consistent with an arterial wound.

On the floor, I am consistent and adamant about the importance of protective gear when handling fluids. In this case, I panicked. I used my bare hands to apply pressure to this man's wound. Blood was just seeping and squirting from between my clenched fingers. I started panicking. One time, we had to do training on 'mass disasters,' where administration brought in dummies with 'wounds' that mimicked wounds sustained during a mass shooting or bombing. I thought I did okay in that training because none of my dummies had 'died,' but now that I was in a real-life situation, I couldn't even speak to the man.

Once a security guard ran down the hall and saw the man was bleeding, he notified the ER and we rushed the patient to a trauma treatment room.

Luckily, the patient only nicked an artery. He did require bullet extraction.

He was arrested for illegal possession by a felon, along with discharging his weapon in public—even though it was a complete accident.

I was treated for first and second-degree burns to my neck and arms, and then I was sent home for the rest of the night—not because I was in trouble, but because I had been involved in a 'traumatic incident.'

Before I could return to work, I had to undergo a mandatory mental health evaluation that is consistent with a Code Silver.

--Y.G.
Nevada

Through Rain, Snow, ER Trips...

I recently read a story in one of your books and was instantly reminded of a somewhat similar incident here.

Someone hit our 'panic' button that is located just outside our emergency room entrance. It is there for patients in such serious condition that they are unable to make it inside, or for patients contaminated with chemicals (those patients are taken straight to a decon room).

As Charge that day, I called for two RNs and we ran up front to see what we were dealing with. The last time someone had hit that button, the patient's arm had been severed in a farming accident. We rarely have anyone hit the button for giggles.

I immediately saw a mailman—in his blue shorts, button-up shirt, and a safari-looking hat—holding up a man I thought could easily be a nightclub bouncer. It was an odd scene, somewhat. The mailman was probably in the 5'2"-5'5" range, while the man he was assisting cleared 6'. The man the mailman was holding up was sobbing loudly.

"What happened?" I asked, as I grabbed a wheelchair and met them in the foyer.

"He's hurt," the mailman replied.

"What happened?" I repeated.

"I don't know," said the mailman. "I knocked on the door, then heard a loud noise. Then, he opened the front door, but he was on the floor. He said he needed a hospital but couldn't afford the ambulance. I have his dog in my truck."

"His dog?" one of my coworkers asked, as she glanced out the window.

"H-help," the injured man cried. "It hurts. It hurts so bad. And my dog, I think he's hurt. Can you help him?"

I know you probably read that as if it all was spoken quickly and coherently, but it was not. It took the patient about three minutes to say those things, and we could hardly understand him.

We couldn't get him to tell us what happened, but he did point to his leg. Right there in the lobby, I rolled up the leg of the man's sweatpants, and wow.

This man's kneecap was dislocated and was pushed nearly to the back of his leg. The area was severely swollen and bruised. It looked as if he had a cantaloupe on his leg.

Once a doctor came in and popped everything back—and the patient received pain medication—he explained that he was excited about a package he'd been expecting, so when he heard the mailman knock, he ran from one end of his home. His dog, a 200-pound mastiff, apparently thought he was playing. The dog ran straight into the patient's knee with his head.

The patient did want us to examine the dog, but our doctor refused. I took the dog from the mailman and gave him a quick once-over, but he appeared fine. Actually, the dog seemed pretty excited to be in a new place and around so many people. We sent RNs out in shifts to stay with the dog in the parking lot.

Our patient still had to leave on crutches, but he wasn't in the critical condition I first assumed when I heard the panic alarm.

One thing's for sure: that patient's mailman sure went the extra mile!

--D.E.
West Virginia

<u>Unfortunate</u>

Mr. Smith had been a frequent flyer for as long as I could remember. We started seeing him when he was in his mid-twenties. He seemed sober each time we saw him, and he answered to using tobacco and alcohol rarely to casually.

The first few times I saw him, I guess I didn't give the visits much thought. He was a young man who worked under the table as a handyman, mostly cutting lawns or helping contractors get jobs finished. His injuries seemed consistent with his line of work.

For example, Mr. Smith first came to our ED because he 'just didn't think' before reaching under a lawnmower to clear a blockage from the blades. Luckily, only one of his fingers required amputation.

Mr. Smith would come in about once a month for work injuries. I guess I would call him a frequent flyer, just because he was a familiar face in our ED, and his injuries were always just severe enough to warrant pain meds and a few hours' worth of 'fix me up,' but usually not severe enough to warrant admission to a floor.

Anyway, Mr. Smith continued seeing us over the years. His visits with us began fluctuating as time passed. There would be times that he'd register two or three times a week, but then we wouldn't see him for three months. Every single visit, though, he'd present with an injury. He never came in for a head cold or anything like that.

Mr. Smith began presenting symptoms of depression in his mid-thirties. We all noticed that he just didn't seem 'right' anymore, and we all reached out to him. He said he'd been involved with several bad relationships and had since given up on his ideal goal of marriage and children. Work was unsteady; he didn't feel comfortable working at a single business, he wanted to continue floating to any available job opening, performing a variety of tasks. He'd been dealing with the loss of his mother, and his home life was nothing spectacular. A doctor suggested that Mr. Smith see a PCP and discuss these feelings. I guess he did, because any other time he visited, he listed an antidepressant as his only regular medication.

It came as quite a shock to us when we heard Mr. Smith's address on the radio as a suicide attempt some five-six years later. He'd still been seeing us regularly. He didn't seem like the most upbeat person in the world, but he didn't seem miserable, either.

Mr. Smith was declared deceased soon after EMS arrived and determined that he had been dead for some time. I guess he called a friend and left a voicemail that stated he was going to kill himself. He asked his friend to call authorities, so his body would not be undiscovered. His friend was traveling and did not receive the voicemail until hours after Mr. Smith had made the call.

What really is shocking about this situation is this: I cannot give you the actual number of times Mr. Smith visited our ED, but I can tell you that in a span of approximately 15 years, we saw him more than 200 times. Like I said, he was prescribed pain medication during most of his visits. Sometimes, he'd been prescribed enough to last 30 days. Other times, he'd been prescribed enough to last five days.

Mr. Smith saved most of those pills throughout the years, and he left a detailed letter that stated he intentionally chose the date of death because of its significance to his 'personal failures.' I guess he'd always had it in his mind that he needed to be married, have a family, and live a certain lifestyle before a certain age, but since he did not attain those things, he committed suicide. We heard he had hundreds of pill bottles filled with medications prescribed by our doctors over the years. Over time, he'd only taken enough to manage his pain. He saved the rest and used them to kill himself, pairing them with his antidepressants and alcohol.

I really can't believe it, even now. I think back to the first time I saw him, and I find myself wondering if he really did have a 15-year suicide plan like he said he did. I beat myself up for not noticing. I know I shouldn't, but I do.

I can only hope that Mr. Smith found peace. I encourage everyone to please reach out to someone—anyone—if they are experiencing these feelings and/or have thoughts of suicide.

--Initials and location withheld at request

Send Nudes

You shared a story from a woman who sent inappropriate pictures to a coworker, when she meant to send them to her spouse. My experience will probably make her feel relieved that this didn't happen to her.

I was fine and dandy owning a flip phone that only had text and phone capabilities, but my husband *insisted* upon purchasing some of these new smart phones. He said we could communicate better with the grandkids, although I know he only wanted the new phones because he wanted to watch football videos on his. The factor in my agreeing to purchase a smart phone was that I could have Facebook access in the palm of my hand, where I have all my work friends and students from nursing school (I teach a class three times per week) on there. My husband helped me set up my accounts, and then he went to work for the night.

On his lunch break, he sent me a text message that said, "Send nudes." It even had a cute winking face.

I made the (very poor) choice to go to the bathroom and strip down to my (very wrinkled) birthday suit and snap a few full-frontal shots for him. I thought I sent them to him.

About ten minutes later, I started receiving notifications from my Facebook account to my e-mail, like 'Jane Smith reacted to your photo on Facebook,' and 'John Smith commented on your photo.'

I used my phone to check my Facebook, and I could have just died.

I uploaded two nude photographs to Facebook. Right under the picture, it had blue text that said, '*Viewed by 201.*' Some people had expressed shock with the 'wow' face under the picture, and two of my male acquaintances from high school commented, 'Looks yummy!' and 'Did you get divorced?'

I tried to delete the pictures, but I couldn't figure out how to do it on the phone, so I hurried to go upstairs to my desktop.

As I was running upstairs, I tripped over my Pomeranian's toy, fell backwards, and I fractured my hip. Thankfully, I still had my new cell phone in my hand, so I called 911.

All I could think about were the pictures, so while I was waiting for an ambulance, I called my husband at work. He was written up for leaving his machine to take the call where I frantically explained how I had uploaded my naked body to social media. I only briefly mentioned hurting my hip.

My husband, bless his heart, turned the whole thing into a joke and said, "Entertaining your boyfriends, huh?"

He said he would leave work and meet me at the hospital, but I told him I was just going to call my sister instead.

When the EMTs arrived, I was still so worked up over the pictures that I asked if they could carry me upstairs to my computer first. They said no.

I was in tears as I explained to two strangers who barely looked old enough to be EMTs what I had done. I sobbed as I told them I *needed* to use my computer, because I couldn't delete the pictures from my phone.

Before they loaded me on the ambulance, one of the EMTs took my phone, saying she could delete the pictures.

She asked, "Do you want to read the comments before I delete them?"

"NO!" I yelled.

She had the pictures deleted in .05 seconds.

I have 1,300 friends on Facebook, and by the time the pictures were deleted, I'm sure most of my friends had seen them.

Thank the Lord, only a handful of people ever mentioned the pictures to me.

My husband got a kick out of the whole situation. It was enough for me to get rid of the smart phone and go back to my flip phone.

--Initials and location withheld at request

<u>Sister Act</u>

Our city has a nunnery, and although it's not what you'd expect to see in movies, the nuns are expected to serve God and follow His laws. It is commonplace to see nuns interacting with our community, but it's somewhat rare to see a nun in our emergency department.

One night, around 02:00, a taxi pulled up and a nun got out. She registered at the desk for vaginal discomfort.

In triage, the Sister told our triage nurse she did not participate in drugs or alcohol, and as a nun, she was not sexually active. Of course, we believed her. Who'd question a nun?!

Well, we were all going on the assumption that the nun had a yeast infection or UTI, something like that.

However, the nun's doctor performed an examination and found discharge and other symptoms consistent with an STD. For a while, the nun went between almost leaving our department to returning to her room to cry. Finally, she consented to an STD test.

It was a mighty shock to discover the nun tested positive for chlamydia.

As soon as she learned she tested positive for an STD, she requested a chapel visit. We paged the appropriate contact for her religion and sent a gentleman in. When he left, it was something out a soap opera. He was literally blotting beads of sweat from his forehead with a silk hanky.

The nun confessed to our doctor that she had been sexually active with a drug dealer. She performed sex willingly, and then she began dabbling in drugs.

This patient begged our doctor and staff not to tell her convent. She was scared that she would be removed. She said she knew what she was doing was wrong in her religion, but she had grown fond of her sexual partner, and she feared she was heading down a dangerous road as far as drugs were concerned. Of course, we couldn't tell anyone if we had wanted to, because of HIPAA.

The doctor prescribed the patient Azithromycin and gave her a pamphlet on addiction. She thanked him, thanked the rest of the staff, and asked if we could call a cab. According to the patient, she had sneaked out to come to our department.

I am just guessing that the patient returned to her residence without being caught. If she was caught, she never returned to our department, at least as far as I am aware.

Since that night, I have always wondered about the people in my life and even those whom I observe but have no real interaction. I guess we are all living lies, whether they're big lies or little ones. It goes to show that not even a nun is perfect.

--R.S.
Indiana

<u>Well...</u>

Back in the late-70s, I was employed as an officer in a rural community that thrived on blue collar work, primarily mining.

I'd say that Jane purchased her house in early-Spring, and we were probably regretting that more than she was.

This lady bought a house that was located about a mile from the primary dig site. The road out in front of her house was a busy one for five to six days a week, from five in the morning to maybe six at night. That particular stretch was also mighty dangerous; plenty of trucks and personal vehicles had run-offs around the curve, which was feet away from Jane's garage. Braking was necessary, usually for anyone going more than 5-10 MPH.

Well, Jane was a complainer. She called our station for *every little thing.* She complained about the machinery noise and mining noise from the dig site. She complained if she saw what she deemed 'too many' vehicles passing through that day. She complained if someone used a foot of her drive way to turn around. She complained if any vehicle had to pull over the grass by the ditch to allow a larger vehicle to pass.

Her biggest complaint, though, drove us bonkers.

Jane did complain about the traffic noise, too, but not nearly as much as she complained about trucks braking.

The calls were endless. This woman would call us two or three times an hour on some days.

"What do you want me to do, Jane?" I remember asking her one day. I was the rookie back then and was usually the one assigned to Jane's calls because nobody else wanted to deal with her.

"I want you to make them stop," she snapped at me.

"I'm not sure I can do that, Jane. That road was there long before your house was. You knew that site was there when you bought the house."

"Well," she yelled, "I didn't know how much noise they'd make."

I was ordered to drive out by Jane's house one day and park my patrol across the street. She actually called that in, too. She said an officer was harassing her, even though I was not near her property, don't think I looked at her house once, and never contacted her. Someone explained to her that I was supposed to be watching the traffic and seeing if trucks were braking unnecessarily. They weren't. And you know what? The noise level wasn't even that bad from where I was sitting. I even had my windows down. I heard one huge slam during my hour there, but the rest of the noise was not too bad. It was definitely not loud enough to disrupt Jane's routine in her home. There were times that I just turned up the radio, and then I couldn't hear the site noise anymore.

I reported to Jane that the noise levels were acceptable, and nobody was braking unnecessarily. Jane was pissed.

She started calling the trucking company, who in turn started calling us. Jane wanted the trucking company to stop driving on that road. The trucking company told us Jane was calling several times per hour, and her calls were disrupting business.

When we went out to pay a visit to Jane, she was standing by the road, painting a message on a piece of plywood. The message said, 'STOP BRAKING BY MY HOME!!!!!!'

A truck drove by while we were approaching Jane. The truck slowed from maybe 30-35 MPH to maybe 7 MPH. There was one brake squeal that lasted maybe a second or so, but otherwise the operation was normal.

Jane flipped out.

We calmed her down and explained that she needed to stop with all the phone calls to the trucking company and to us. The guys were well within their rights, and they were not braking excessively.

This didn't stop Jane's behavior. We got a call one day that Jane had marched down to the dig site and picketed. She wanted the drivers to stop braking in front of her home, and she wanted the dig site to close.

By the time we arrived to the site, Jane was back at home. I felt bad for the guys who'd just put up with her, because she was a firecracker when I arrived. At one point, I thought I'd have to arrest her. We didn't want to have to do that. Arresting someone in our community was a big to-do. We tried to give everyone multiple opportunities to correct their behavior. That worked for us back then.

It was the next day that crap hit the fan.

Jane had placed 100 calls to the trucking company in two hours, and they were fed up with her nonsense.

We responded to Jane's frantic call and were shocked at what we witnessed.

The trucking company's boss went out to the dig site and personally drove one of his trucks back. This time, though, he followed Jane's demand to not brake.

This 7,000-pound dump truck that was carrying a measly 10 short tons of gravel plowed right went around that curve at roughly 15 MPH, left the road, and plowed right through Jane's garage. It left her vehicle totaled, and it brought the whole garage down.

The driver was uninjured and still in the vehicle when I arrived. He said he 'accidentally' unloaded the gravel he was carrying at the edge of Jane's yard. My partner asked him to get out of the truck, and I was on Jane-duty.

Jane managed to get away from me and she rushed toward the truck driver.

"You ruined my property!" she screamed. "Do you have any idea how much I paid for that car?"

The owner of the company shrugged and said, "Well, you told us to stop braking."

"So, you just thought you'd come in my yard? You could have turned the other way."

The guy said, "Turn the other way? Are you nuts? I would've killed myself. Just imagine if that truck was one of my guys carrying a full load, or if they didn't know how to handle a run-off like I do."

Jane wanted to press charges, but we listed the incident as a traffic accident and cited the owner/driver for not braking. The company's insurance paid for Jane's garage and her vehicle. Their truck was not damaged, except for a few dings.

Jane was pissed that she'd lost the fight, so she listed the house just a few months after she'd bought it. None of us thought she'd get what she paid for it. We heard rumors that she would probably sell at only 75-80% of what she originally had paid.

Unfortunately, Jane was coming back from the city and learned first-hand about that road and the importance of braking. She admitted to us that she didn't slow down, so she hit a patch of ice, plowed down her mail box, spun back on the road, and hit a tree head-on. *One of the truckers saw the whole thing unfold, and he called in the accident. He stayed with her until EMS and our guys arrived, so she wouldn't be scared.* She was taken to the hospital for a broken arm and broken neck.

Jane took her house off the market after her accident, and she never called us again. She even sent the trucker who'd stayed with her flowers and a thank you card. I'm sorry that it had to come to all that, but at least it didn't end as badly as it could have. I'm not saying that the truck driver was right in what

he did, but he tried to teach her a lesson.
Apparently, though, it was a lesson she had to
learn on her own.

--D.T.
West Virginia

You're Right, You Win

I am a little person with skeletal dysplasia, and I stand proud at three-foot-one. I am a registered nurse on Pediatrics, and I love my job. I feel that children respond well to my size, so it makes 'not fun' things like IV insertion easier. A lot of my kids are between the ages of two and eight, so I think they see me as 'one of them' and it makes for happier patients and happier nurses.

I was freaking out one night because I had lost my ring. My boyfriend had proposed to me the night before, and I was in the middle of a 12- hour shift when I looked down and realized the ring wasn't on my finger.

Man, I searched everywhere for that ring. I crawled under beds, tore through the linen closet, moved everything off the counters…You name a place, and I can guarantee that I frantically looked there a billion times.

Finally, it hit me: I had gone out to my car and on the way back in, I had helped one of our housekeepers unload her trash bin to the dumpster.

Well, I told my coworker that I'd be back, but I didn't tell her what I was doing.

I went outside and climbed up on a stack of pallets. I lifted the heavy dumpster lid and was hanging over the side of the huge bin, using the light on my cell phone to look inside. It was mostly empty, except for the trash I'd helped the housekeeper toss.

My arm was getting tired of holding the lid open, and my stomach was hurting because I had to lay over the edge of the bin to be able to see into it, so I kind of wiggled around to get more comfortable.

Right as I saw my ring at the bottom of the bin, I fell in. The lid slammed shut behind me.

I could tell I was hurt right away, but I didn't know how bad it was. My ankle felt like someone had hit me with a baseball bat, and my shoulder hurt. It was dark in the dumpster, and it reeked, of course. I couldn't reach the lid, and no matter how I tried, I couldn't climb out. I could feel stuff squirming under my hands as I steadied myself, and I'd somehow lost one of my shoes, so my sock was soaked.

I started panicking because I couldn't find my phone. Just a few seconds later, I heard it ringing. I had dropped my phone outside of the bin.

I yelled for help, but I knew I didn't have much of a chance at anyone hearing me. Only the housekeepers and our nurses really used that exit, and the housekeepers were done on that side of the hospital. The only nurse who'd come out to smoke recently did so, and she only came out once every four hours.

I was panicking. For some reason, since my boyfriend made me watch *Star Wars,* I've always had this irrational fear that I'd be stuck in a trash compactor. Well, here I was, trapped in a dumpster. I started freaking out over the irrational fear that there was some kind of monster in the bin with me. Then, I started thinking that the walls were going to close in on me.

My coworker, thankfully, noticed I had been gone an unusually long amount of time, so she reported my absence to the Nursing

Supervisor. The NS activated a code, in which two people from each floor are supposed to stop what they are doing and search the grounds for the missing person. It's really in case patients go missing or someone had a medical emergency, you know, like in case someone passed out in one of the bathrooms that nobody ever goes to.

Someone came outside and found my shoe and phone. They called out my name, and I started screaming my head off.

"Oh my gosh," this woman exclaimed, as she lifted the bin lid and saw me. "How did you get in there?"

I told her to get me out of there, and then I would tell her.

She reached down and told me to grab her hand. She tried to pull me up, and my shoulder popped. I didn't care; I wasn't letting go, even if it killed me.

The NS sent me to ES and I was first sent to the decontamination area to bathe because I was covered in maggots and what I still call 'trash juice.' Then, I was treated for a dislocated shoulder, a laceration to my other shoulder, and a sprained ankle. I was given a week off work to recuperate. My boyfriend's (now husband's) mom stayed at our apartment to help me do stuff around the house, like clean and take care of our pug.

So, I've read a lot of your stories and stories about people having bad days, and I just wanted to share my own. I can laugh about it now, but that was such a bad shift that I think I'm in the running with some of the stuff I've read.

--J.R.-W.
New York

<u>Bright Idea</u>

My partner and I were the first medics on scene, to an explosion that occurred some three decades ago. The scene was grisly.

When we arrived, we found four injured males. One male was in such bad shape that it was obvious that he was deceased. The other three males suffered from injuries that ranged in severity to minor to critical. Their injuries included burns and shrapnel embedded in their bodies. One male had a piece of metal, approximately four-inches in length, jutting out from his chest. He complained of shortness of breath, heaviness in his chest, and—surprise—chest pain.

I can't go into detail about the rest of the injuries or what happened on scene, but three more buses arrived, and the coroner was notified. Law enforcement followed us to the hospital, where they interviewed the remaining explosion victims.

Apparently, one of the teenagers wondered what would happen if the group placed explosives in a pressure cooker. One male then took his family's pressure cooker to a shed behind another friend's home. Another teen stole ammunition and gun powder from his father's ammunition storage.

The teenagers huddled inside a shed that was no larger than the bathroom in my apartment. I'd say that the teens were no further than three to five feet away from the pressure cooker when it exploded.

Only one victim passed away that day. The male with the shrapnel poking out from his chest survived. I was informed the metal missed his aorta by less than a quarter of an inch. The other males were forced to live with the scars for the rest of their lives, on top of the guilt and traumatic memories stemming from this event.

I don't know what the kids were thinking would happen, to be honest. Common sense would tell us that mixing pressure and high temps with ammunition would not provide a good result, but I also remember being young and doing stupid things.

This is one call that I have never been able to shake from my mind because I've always

wondered, 'Why? Why would you do that?
Why would you do that in a confined area?
Why would you think this would go any other
way?'

--Initials and location withheld at request

<u>Updates</u>

I saw you post that you often have to dig through 'bad' submissions that revolve around sad stories before you find 'good' submissions, so I thought I would share one of the 'good' ones.

My story starts off as a bad one. I have been a nurse on PICU for 40 years. I've seen it all, and my heart has broken a million times.

I cared for baby Jane from birth. She was not expected to live more than 48 hours. She was a fighter, though, so 48 hours became 72, which became a month, and so on.

Finally, when Jane was eight-months-old, she was released to her family. Unfortunately, she still required a great deal of medical care, as she had a g-tube, trach tube, and she was on a vent. She returned to my unit a week after her release, and she stayed with us until she was 14-months. She was then released again. Doctors said that Jane would likely pass away before her next birthday. Her family moved out of state, and I never heard about Jane again.

Well, a few months ago, I received a friend request on Facebook. I did not recognize the woman by her picture or name, so I denied the request.

Two days later, she sent another. Again, I denied the request.

The next day, she'd sent yet *another* request. I was starting to feel that I needed to block her. Who was this insane lady? Was she a scammer? We didn't have mutual friends on Facebook, so she couldn't have added me from a friend's profile. It was driving me bonkers.

My granddaughter was messing with my phone and she said, "Nana, some woman is sending you a chat request."

"Ignore it," I said. I was cooking dinner and watching the news, so I was a little distracted.

"But Nana," she told me, "I already hit yes. She said you took care of some baby. Jane. Should I say anything back?"

I dropped my cooking spoon so fast that it fell off the counter. My dog wasted no time rushing over, grabbing the spoon, and running off with it in his mouth. (That's why I call him 'The Vulture.' He's always watching you, circling you, if he thinks you have food.)

The woman messaging me and sending me friend requests was Jane's mother.

Jane is now attending college and is engaged to be married. She was a 4.0 student and received a full scholarship to a prestigious nursing program.

I cannot tell you how long I cried after hearing that news and seeing photographs of Jane all grown up.

There are happy endings out there, despite what the media and everyone else would like you to believe. Miracles happen every day, and good news comes when you least expect it. I hope you and your readers can remember this story when you're feeling that there is no good left in the world. I know good news exists because my patient beat the odds and proved all those doctors wrong. She's now a healthy, happy adult. I could not be prouder of my profession, and I'm also proud that Jane was such a fighter.

--S.M.
Maine

V.I.P.

I recently quit my job based on what I felt to be unethical practices. This is the incident that pushed me over the edge.

We were short-staffed and busy as busy could be. We were all overloaded with too many patients, but administration didn't seem to care. We were not allowed to call in extra help, so we were each assigned between four to nine patients throughout the shift.

I was somehow expected to care for five patients *and* do triage at the same time. Three of my patients were in stable condition and were admitted to our ER for things such as non-symptomatic ETOH counseling or migraines. Two of my patients were admitted for things like diabetes complications or tachycardia.

The waiting room was packed. Our registration clerks were both in tears as they battled irritated and impatient patients, all while answering a bombardment of phone calls.

Most of the patients in the waiting room were complaining of actual emergencies. For example, one patient had a knife sticking out from his abdomen. We simply did not have an open room to place him.

A woman arrived in the ER, escorted by her husband. They were both dressed in designer clothes and had a smugness that surrounded them.

I was about to call another patient to triage as the woman demanded to the one registration clerk, "Get me a room right now. I think I have broken my finger."

"I can certainly get you registered, ma'am," said the registration clerk. "We see patients on a severity of injury basis, so you will first be triaged based on the severity of your complaint, and then you will be called back based on the severity of your injury."

"I said get me a room. I didn't say sit there and argue with me," the woman snapped.

"Ma'am," I said sternly, "this clerk is correct. Please check in and have a seat. I do have a few people in front of you, but I will absolutely call you to triage as soon as possible, and we will do all we can to have you treated as soon as we have rooms available."

"Do you know who I am?" the woman shouted at me. "I am the reason you have this job."

"That may be," I replied. "But, we have rules in place for the protection of *all* patients. If you required immediate intervention, we certainly would not call back someone with a broken finger. I promise, as soon as we can get you to a treatment area, we will."

I called the next patient to triage, while the woman was still at the front, pitching a fit. She demanded her husband get her cell phone from her purse.

I triaged three patients and assisted in sending one of my patients to Cath Lab and securing placement for another patient to a rehab center for his alcohol dependence. As I was dialing to ICU to find a bed for another patient, someone came up to my work area and pressed on my phone, effectively ending my call.

"Excuse me," I said with a huff.

"Who do you think you are, to tell one of our valued contributors that she will have to wait for treatment?"

I stared up at the hospital CEO.

I said to him, "I simply explained that we treat patients based on the severity of the complaints."

"No," he shouted. "You don't make someone like Mrs. Smith wait. She has been out in that lobby for twenty-six minutes, thanks to you and your incompetence. That is unacceptable."

Everyone was staring at me, even patients. I have never been so embarrassed in my life! I was about to cry, but my defense mechanism kicked in, and I became angry instead.

"We seated a stab victim for an hour and a half," I exclaimed. "I didn't see you coming down here to fight for *him* to be seen sooner."

The CEO turned bright red and told me I was out of line. He asked me, "And, that stab victim didn't donate a million dollars to our facility, did he?"

I asked, "So, what you're saying is that you have to give the hospital money to be treated properly?"

The CEO refused to answer my question and threatened to have my license revoked.

I walked out, right there in the middle of my shift.

While I worked in that hospital, I can't tell you how many hypocrites I encountered. These people are the first to bash online bloggers who complain about work, but apparently, it's perfectly acceptable to make fun of the patient while the patient is still in the ER. It's perfectly fine to leave your post so you can have sex with a married man, but it's not okay to use the restroom or take coffee to a worried family.

This situation made me feel angry beyond words.

I did not join the healthcare industry to discriminate against patients in any way. In nursing school, all I heard was 'don't judge,' and for the most part, I try not to. Admittedly, I have some of the same thoughts you and other readers have, but that never affects patient care. I can think that you are an idiot, but I will not treat you as if you are less important because of what you did. I was floored to hear in not so many words that this facility valued a benefactor's monetary contributions over the life of someone suffering from a true emergency.

I have only been an RN for three years, so I know I am relatively new, but I really hope I'm not going to encounter things like this all my life.

--Initials and location withheld at request

After examining a 4-year-old, I asked my nurse, "Can you get him scheduled for a T & A?"

The patient's mother gasped and angrily scolded, "I hardly think that's appropriate. He's only a kid, and I don't know how that would help his sore throat. After I report you, you'll never be able to get a job again."

I then had to explain that I did *not* wish to schedule her son for what adults know to be 'T & A,' but that in the medical world, 'T & A' meant tonsillectomy and adenoidectomy.

Geez.

--M.K., M.D.
Maryland

What Were You Thinking?

Our newest RN was truly *new*. She'd been an RN for three months. When you're new to the ER, you're full of life, idealistic, and are vulnerable to emotions that many of us have learned to manage to save our own lives.

Jane came to me one night. It was during summer, and we were about to discharge a homeless patient who'd come in after a fight. Jane was sobbing when she told me that she 'just couldn't' send the patient back to the streets. She had tried to find him housing, but no shelter would take him due to his violent history and being kicked out of every shelter in the area.

"Honey," I said, "you can't save everyone. I know it's hard, but some people have to try to help themselves, and you have to let them."

Jane sniffled a little bit. I had no doubt that Jane's patient was taking her on a guilt trip and leading her to a pity party. After all, he'd done it to all of us. His story always changed. It was everyone else's fault that he was in the position that he was in. The shelter administrators were bad people because they wouldn't let him do drugs in the bathroom. They were horrible people because they kicked him out after he attacked a pregnant woman. It wasn't *his* fault that he was busted for attempted rape or a mugging. He actually said to me, "If that bitch hadn'ta screamed so loud, the cop wouldn'tve come to check on her."

One time, John told our Charge that it was the hospital's responsibility to rent homeless people apartments. When we told him that we could only offer the numbers for shelters or call a few for him, he reacted violently and broke a tech's arm. He had shelter that night: jail. But, thanks to overcrowding, he was back on the street. He was never held more than a few weeks at a time.

Well, Jane went off to discharge the patient and was gone for a few minutes longer than usual. I figured the patient was giving her grief, so I went to the lobby to check on her. She and the patient were all smiles as he departed, and I saw him carrying a wad of cash.

"Did you give him money?" I exclaimed.

"He needed a cab," she said with a shrug.

Maybe it was the bitter old hag in me, but I just shook my head and thought to myself, 'Is that what they're calling drugs these days?'

Jane was in high spirits for a while, and some of us thought this was unusual, just because she had spent most of her time with us bawling about everything. None of us got on her about that because we knew what it was like to be new. I guess it's true, that the longer you've been doing this, you get kind of jaded. You realize that some people live and some die. You tell yourself that there's really nothing else you could have done, that when it's someone's time, it's their time. You can get someone help, but if they are unwilling to help themselves, you'll see them a thousand more times. So, we were glad to see that Jane was happy. We thought that maybe she was coming to terms with not being able to single-handedly save the world like most young nurses dream of when they enter the program.

"Hey," I called down to her, "some of us are going out for drinks after this shift, going to grab some pizza, too. Do you want to come?"

She smiled and replied, "Thanks, but I told John I would make him dinner."

"I didn't think you were seeing anyone," another coworker said.

She shook her head. "I'm not."

"John," she said, pointing to the room where the homeless patient had been. "I gave him my extra house key and told him to take a cab. He's going to shower, and then I'm going to make him dinner when I get home."

At first, we were all silent. Then, we started chuckling.

"You got us," I said. "You really had me going there for a second."

Jane looked confused. "I wasn't kidding. I'm making chicken parmigiana. I told him he could live with me as long as he wanted."

We started bombarding Jane with things like, "Are you crazy?" and "What if he murders you?"

Our Charge felt like he had no other choice but to notify our Supervisor. In turn, she notified HR and Risk Management because a boundary had been violated. She then notified the police, but they said they couldn't do anything because Jane *wanted* the patient to stay. Even the officers were familiar with John and told Jane what a bad idea this was, but she stood her ground. Oh, it was nuts during all that. The Supervisor even pulled Jane from her other patients and took her upstairs to discuss how serious this was. Jane didn't care.

When we realized that Jane wasn't budging on her decision, a few of us finally convinced her to invite us to dinner, too. We wanted to make sure she wasn't going to walk in her house and get beheaded or something, or that John wouldn't stab her while she was cooking. Another guy offered to stay the night and sleep on the couch, just to make sure she was safe during the night, but Jane acted offended that any of us even had the thought that John would hurt her.

After our shift ended, we all loaded up in a coworker's car and followed Jane home. I can't even repeat some of the things that we said in the car because all of us have watched too much I.D. TV and were talking about all the scenarios that could unfold. It was exciting and terrifying at the same time.

When we got to Jane's house and all got out of the car, Jane was freaking out because her front door was wide open, and we could see some stray dogs running in and out with her shoes and the throw pillows she kept on her couch.

Okay, that couldn't be a good sign.

We heard sirens as we approached the house. One of the guys with us told Jane not to go inside, that he would go in and make sure John was gone. While he was inside, Jane's neighbor came over and said she called the police because she noticed a strange man coming in and out of her house.

Officers arrived, and once we determined John was not in the house, we followed Jane inside.

The mess. Oh dear, the mess.

Jane's dishwasher and washing machine had been filled with who-knows-how-much detergent, and both had overflowed. Bubbles oozed out of Jane's kitchen/laundry room area and were all over her living room floor. Furniture was turned over. We flipped her couch to its upright position and had to wash our hands because the couch was covered in urine and it looked like John took a knife to the cushions. Most of Jane's electronics were still there, except for the small stuff, like her tablet. All her jewelry was gone. Jane was in tears because John had broken a piggy bank that been passed through her family since the early-1900s, and he took all the money inside. There were holes in most of her walls, and her toilet had been cracked. John clogged Jane's tub and sink, so they both flooded and the carpet in Jane's hallway was soaked and ruined. I don't know why, but my coworker opened Jane's fridge...John defecated in the refrigerator and took most of her food.

The weirdest part of John's thievery was that he took all her undergarments, and I mean all of them. He took a few of her clothes, too, and she noticed some of her luggage was missing.

Officers found John downtown that night. He was handing out Jane's underwear and bras to prostitutes and had traded some of her jewelry for drugs. He had one of Jane's rolling suitcases that he'd filled with food. Jane said one of the officers found one of her Scentsy warmers and a Glade plug-in in the suitcase, but it made no sense why he'd take things like that.

We didn't see John for a long time after that because he went to jail. He eventually got sent to prison, but not for what he did to Jane's house.

Jane had a nightmare of a time with her insurance company. They tried to argue that she was responsible for the damages because she allowed someone in her home. I don't know exactly how she got them to pay, but they covered most of the damages. She stayed with a coworker for a while, until she could get her locks changed and get people out to repair the toilet and stuff.

At work, Jane was reprimanded for violating patient/caretaker boundaries. I don't think it was severe, though, because administration can't really control everything you do outside of the hospital. I think she was mostly in trouble because she was on duty when this happened.

Though the events were unfortunate, I'd say it's safe to say that Jane learned her lesson. I'm just glad she wasn't injured.

--Y.P.
California

The Day the Comments Section Came to Life

We were dispatched to a rural farming supply store for a complaint of a middle-age male being destructive and combative. When we arrived, this male had stripped down to his skivvies and was eating popcorn by the handful, straight out of the popcorn machine. He was heavily intoxicated. What's more is that this male was an employee at the store. Coworkers gave statements that this subject had been 'down' lately and had been talking about quitting his job 'in a big way.' This was his way, apparently, to get plastered on shift, remove all his clothing, ride child-sized bicycles around the store, knock over clothing racks, empty candy bins on the floors, and end his wild streak by hitting up the popcorn machine. Obviously, he was taken in custody.

Someone in our community set up a Facebook page, and on that page, most of our scanner feed is posted for public awareness.

This has been largely helpful in keeping busybodies at home, rather than crowded around a scene. This has also been annoying, as I will explain.

On this day, someone posted about the situation with the drunk subject. If you are familiar with the Facebook comments section, I need not explain because you will probably already know what kind of drama seeps from the comments. However, if you are not familiar with the comments section of Facebook, allow me to explain. Apparently, everyone posting comments has a degree in law enforcement, substance abuse/rehabilitation, animal welfare, child welfare, traffic laws, and just about any other topic you can imagine. You cannot post a simple opinion, because then you will have 15,000 people ganging up on you, calling you names, telling you why you are wrong. I have even seen outrageous comments on simple pictures. For example, my neighbor posted a picture of her dog lying on her king-size bed. People ganged up on this woman, saying things like, "You don't deserve a dog," and "Someone should come and shoot you for how you treat that poor animal. Why did you get a dog, if you don't take care of him?" They said these things because the dog was missing a leg. My neighbor rescued this dog, who was missing a leg because his previous owners left the dog outside, where he became caught in a metal chain for so long that he, as a large breed dog, weighed 10-pounds at a year old, and his leg had essentially died. This dog is treated like royalty, yet all these people joined an angry virtual mob to hate on her picture of this dog lying on her $2,000 bed.

This is what happened in the comments section on the post about the drunk subject. Some patients were cracking jokes about the situation. Yes, while it was sad that the subject's life had taken such a bad turn, some of the jokes were funny. If you can't see the light in these situations, I don't know what else to tell you, other than have fun with your 'that's not funny' life. Anyway, other comments were of concern for the subject's wellbeing and prayers that he found his way to a 12-step program (to which someone replied, "Judging by what I heard on the scanner, it doesn't sound like he can even take two steps without falling down.").

Shortly after the initial post was made, keyboard warriors began arguing with each other in the comments section, much like I explained happened to my neighbor's picture of her dog. There were people threatening each other, calling each other names, and you couldn't have an opinion on the matter either way because from one side, people would be coming at you and saying you were heartless, while on the other side, people would be coming at you and saying you weren't funny. We were made aware of these comments because someone actually called our station to report them.

Yes, someone *called the police department* to report, "Hey, you know that guy you just arrested? People are making fun of him on Facebook."

Really? Quick, sound the alarm! Put out a bulletin to arrest every last commenter with dark humor!

We monitored the comments, and we even saw our caller posted her own comment that read, "For all you people mocking this man, just know that the cops were called. They're watching you, and they're going to arrest you now."

I have to admit, I got a good chuckle out of that one.

We noticed that two commenters started calling each other out to meet in real life, and within a matter of minutes, two became six. This also occurs from time to time in the comments section, but people don't usually show. We figured it couldn't hurt to go down to the place they were challenging each other to meet at. If nobody showed up, great. If they did show up, yay (we need a sarcasm font).

We drove across town and saw a bunch of people fighting in the Burger King parking lot. My partner and I knew immediately that we needed backup, because there weren't just a few people there…I guessed there were about 15 people brawling and a whole bunch more watching the fight go down.

The department sent all available units to the parking lot, where subjects were fighting with baseball bats, fists, and one man— obviously the brightest and most prepared one there—came armed with a replica sword and homemade chain mail armor.

Boy, we were busy, busy, busy for a few hours, processing all these arrests, dealing with checking for warrants (yep, we nabbed a few brawlers who were running from the law), all that fun stuff. Surprisingly, only two subjects received medical treatment. I guess everyone else just went about slapping each other. Big talkers on the computer, but not one person there sustained anything more than a superficial laceration.

And, wouldn't you know it, not only did the fight make it to a post on Facebook, but the bust of the fighting ring also had its own post. I think there were about 400 comments on that one, just about an hour after it had been posted, and it was eventually removed because idiots were on there, challenging each other to another fight! I guess you can't fix stupid.

There is great news with this story, by the way. Our original subject, John, caught wind that all these extra people were in jail because they were fighting about a post made about his drunken actions. John was mortified and after serving his time, he completed inpatient rehab at a nearby facility. He's been in AA ever since, and I don't think he's had a relapse. We've touched base with him a few times, usually while he's been doing his court-ordered community service, and John has accredited the Facebook post to showing him how much trouble he'd gotten himself into and for embarrassing him so much that he knew he needed to quit drinking and stay sober.

We still monitor that Facebook page, but we haven't had to break up any brawls stemming from comments since that day.

--H.E.
Tennessee

The Hunt

I am a long-time faithful reader, but I have to admit this: as I was reading the first few of your books, I found myself a little skeptical of some of the stories that took place. I thought to myself, 'Nobody could ever possibly do something *that* stupid.' I mean, I have worked in ES for almost a decade, and I couldn't relate to any of the absurd chief complaints or injuries. (I could, however, relate to the rude patients and families.) I was baffled because I started reading your reader-submitted stories, and I wondered what the heck kind of hospitals these people work at; I guess our ES is just quiet.

It wasn't until recently that my mind changed, and I realized firsthand how some people do ridiculous things.

I was up front, trying to get change from the registration girl, when a woman walked up to the registration counter. I shouldn't say she 'walked,' because what she did was more of a waddle, as if she had a groin injury or something of the sort. Registration couldn't open the cash drawer until the patient was taken care of, so I just stood in the corner with my money, and I watched this woman explain why she was there.

"My boyfriend was gone all day," she said calmly. "He went to take his kids to an Easter egg hunt."

"Okay…?" the registration girl said.

"I wanted to surprise him."

My mind started roaming to the possibility that the woman penetrated herself too deeply with a toy or something. Then, I started rationalizing that she did say she wanted to surprise him, so then I started thinking that maybe she tried to Nair off her pubic hair and received a chemical burn. I was also thinking about how slowly this was going, because I was expecting the delivery man at any second, and I knew he wouldn't have change for a twenty.

"We were going to have our own egg hunt," the woman continued.

An elderly couple entered the lobby and stood behind the woman. I heard them bickering about lab orders.

"So," she said, with no visible embarrassment or shame "you know those plastic eggs that you can get from Wal-Mart? Well, I got some of them, and I thought it would be fun to make him find them, but now we can't get them out."

I thought, 'No way.'

"Out of where?" the registration girl asked.

"I have two down there," she pointed to her vagina and then to her buttocks, "and one back there."

"Oh, honey!" the old woman behind her exclaimed, "Why on Earth would you do something like that?"

I couldn't help but to laugh, and I think it was just at the sight of the elderly woman's concerned and bewildered facial expression.

"We thought they'd come out," she shrugged.

I cannot stress enough how this woman talked like this was something commonplace.

She did not seem to care *at all* what anyone else thought.

"Did you try to push them out?" the elderly man asked. "Because that's how hens lay eggs. You have to push real hard, and your body does the rest of the work. That's how ladies have babies."

"Hush, John," his wife said. She slapped him in the chest with her pocketbook.

I had to run to the triage room and was doubled over in laughter. I was trying to hide it by burying my face in a stack of towels, but I'm sure the patient and the elderly couple heard me.

"Uh," the registration girl stammered, "so, uh, you have a foreign body in your rectum and vagina. Okay…Uh…I need your name."

This poor girl was so confused that she could barely piece together a sentence, which made me laugh even harder.

I guess it was instant karma for laughing so much, because I was the one assigned to the patient.

The egg in her rectum was somewhat difficult to dislodge for two reasons. Firstly, the patient had used a liberal amount of lubricant to place the egg in her rectum. This made it difficult to grab. Secondly, the patient had had stuffed the plastic egg with 'treats.' In this case, she placed a small packet of flavored heat-activated lubrication in the egg. In our attempt to dislodge the egg, it opened, and the plastic edging tore the thin film containing the lubrication. The patient started breathing heavily and squirming because she said she could feel the lube heating up and it was 'burning [her] insides.' It took 20 minutes to remove that egg, and by the time the procedure was done, the patient was crying and begging for the burning to stop. The doctor ordered an enema to try to flush the excess lubricant because she rated her pain an eight out of ten.

We returned to the room about twenty minutes later, and we tried to dislodge the eggs from the woman's vaginal cavity.

Of course, the doctor's first instruction to the patient was to push, which was a horrible idea, following an enema. Feces basically squirted and leaked to the floor. I was disgusted, but our doc had history on L & D, so he didn't even seem to notice. Instead, he told her to push again. The woman grunted and cried, citing a pinching sensation.

Upon closer examination, the doctor realized that, somehow, the eggs had opened and partially closed upon one another and her cavity wall. She suffered from minimal vaginal bleeding.

We kept the patient until she had another bowel movement, and we sent her packing afterward.

You know, if I would have read this story in one of your books, I would have been skeptical. I know it happens now, though, because it happened to me. I've been re-reading your books with more of an open mind, especially after seeing something like this in person.

--U.E.
Illinois

I have lost count on how many complaints of 'green poop' I encounter in the days following St. Patrick's Day. As a physician having to explain food coloring to men and women ranging in age from 18-45, I find myself increasingly concerned about the direction of our species.

--B.E., M.D.
North Carolina

They'll Repeat Everything

I am a school nurse in an elementary school for children in grades Pre-K through third.

One day, a teacher's assistant knocked on my door. She was holding the hand of a little boy no older than five years old, and when it came time to speak, she was laughing so hard that tears streamed down her cheeks.

"Tell her what you told me," she said to the boy.

"I need to use a vibrator," he said, confused as to why his teacher was laughing.

"Uh…," I said.

"My head hurts," he said. "I need to use a vibrator."

The teacher's assistant was laughing so hard that she had to sit down.

"Why do you say that?" I asked.

"Because when my mom says her head hurts, my dad says he can help her with that, but my mom says she'll use her vibrator," he said innocently.

I could barely contain myself as I made the phone call to his mother, explaining what he said and that he had a low-grade fever.

When his mom came to pick him up, she could barely look me in the eye. She embarrassingly assured me that she would have a talk with her son.

--E.M.-K.
Michigan

I'm Telling

I am a retired medic and my husband is a retired K-9 officer. We firmly believe in using surveillance equipment to protect our property, and I can't recall a time in our married lives that we haven't kept a trained German Shepherd. My grandkids joke that Nana and Papa's home is 'like a prison' because of all our cameras, the padlock on our fence, and all the signs we have up about surveillance and no trespassing.

One night, I was in the kitchen, preparing my medications while my husband was getting our late-night movie started. I noticed that the dogs were acting anxious, so I opened the door to let them patrol the yard. They bolted as soon as the door was open, and I knew something was wrong.

Before I could step foot on the patio, I heard someone scream, and then I heard the fence rattle. I yelled for my husband to call the police, and I went to check on the dogs. I didn't see anyone in my yard or the neighbors' yards.

My husband told me to go inside with our older dog, and he went out with a flashlight and our younger dog. I was watching our security monitors and saw a man approach my yard while my husband was by our storage shed. My older dog ran to the back door and barked, and I could see on the monitor that the younger dog was doing the same in the yard. I heard my husband shout, and on the monitor, I could see the man run away.

My husband found a syringe filled with drugs just inside our yard, so when the police arrived, he handed it over to officers. They said they would add an extra patrol to the neighborhood for the night, but they said the man was probably aware that he could not come back because he knew we had dogs.

We left the dogs in the yard for about an hour, just for peace of mind. We never heard them bark, and I never saw anything suspicious on the cameras, so we brought the dogs in and went to bed.

I think we were asleep for about thirty to forty minutes, when there was a furious pounding on our front door. It was the type of pounding you would expect when someone was trying to break in your home or when you lock an angry person out.

My husband loaded his gun and told me to call the police again. He made the dogs stay in our bedroom, and he told me to lock the bedroom door and not let him in unless he said our emergency 'password.'

Without access to our security cameras, I was a nervous wreck. I didn't know what was going on, but I knew that no good could come from someone beating on the door after midnight. Dispatch informed me officers were on the way. When I told her my husband was armed, she dispatched additional units. I always thought it was funny, that when you say you're armed, officers make it a special point to get there a little bit quicker, as opposed to saying nobody is armed. My husband always said it's because situations tend to escalate quicker than when both parties are unarmed.

Downstairs, I could hear glass breaking and things crashing around. There are no words to express how I felt when I heard a gunshot. The dogs were going crazy, and I was hiding in the closet, sobbing as I stayed on the line with the 911 operator. I had no idea if my husband was injured—or worse—dead.

Officers arrived, and I heard my husband call up to me that it was safe to come out. I left the dogs in our bedroom as I went downstairs.

Officers had two males in custody. One male, I identified as the person I saw on the security camera. In person, it was clear that he was still a teenager, probably not even old enough to have graduated high school. The other male was probably in his mid-40s.

The teenager had entered our yard because he thought he could shoot up in our shed. He dropped his drugs when the dogs chased him out of the yard. He tried to come back for the drugs before the police arrived the first time (when the dogs barked the second time). He didn't know that my husband had turned the drugs over to the police department. I guess the teenager came back after he noticed all our lights were off, and he searched our yard for his syringe. When he couldn't find it, he went home and told his dad that we'd stolen his drugs.

Father of the year drove to our house to confront us. He demanded that my husband return the drugs. When my husband told them (through the locked screen door) to leave, the two punched through the screen door and a scuffle ensued. The noises I heard were my hall table being knocked over and my decorative water basin being smashed. My husband fired a warning shot (he said he didn't want to shoot anyone, so he gave them the opportunity to leave). Police officers pulled up as the two intruders were running to their car. Both were arrested on multiple charges.

It is truly a crazy world we're living in right now!

--A.Y.
Virginia

The Blind Leading the Blind

I work on ICU, and just like ER RNs, we also see frequent flyers. On this day, Mr. Smith was admitted for an overdose. It was his sixth OD in only a few months, and it was also his sixth stay on our unit.

Each time Mr. Smith was admitted, his friends would stop by. His friends were also addicts, so when they would arrive to visit him, they were always drunk or high. We always had to call security and/or law enforcement to escort them from the property, due to their behavior.

This day, I think everyone in the hospital felt overwhelmed. We were short-staffed, and all day, we'd been hearing that other departments were as well. Mr. Smith's friends were not making working on our floor any easier.

For starters, it was obvious John was hammered. He could hardly stand. His friend, James, also appeared to be under the influence of drugs.

When John fell and broke the waiting room coffee table, we called security. The call rang back to switchboard, and the operator told us all guards were busy with police and firefighters, as there was a gas leak in one of the older wings. Switchboard said she would connect me with the police department.

As I was waiting to connect, our emergency alarms sounded, and a message came over the intercom system that ordered all personnel to activate evacuation protocol. All visitors were instructed to leave the property in an orderly manner. As far as I am aware, the facility never had a real evacuation before that day. We'd only received training via seminars, and a year earlier, all personnel had to attend a 15-minute training seminar to use Evac-Chairs, which are chairs where you place non-ambulatory patients, strap them in, and two staff members move this chair down steps—one person stands behind the patient, while another lifts from the patient's feet, all while the patient is in a seated position.

Of course, all attention was on patients. We are on the fourth floor, and during an evacuation, elevators stop operating. On ICU that day, we had nine non-ambulatory patients and three patients capable of following evacuation procedure. We only had three nurses, though, and it would take all three of us to transfer patients to the Evac-Chair, and then two of us to carry the patients down the steps.

We tried to use the paging system to call for all available personnel to assist us in evacuating patients, but other floors were doing the same thing, so the paging system crashed. One of my coworkers literally ran up two flights of stairs and back down, with two orderlies she was able to catch before they could make it to a floor to help. She had pleaded with them and explained that there was simply no way that three RNs (especially one of us who was 16-weeks pregnant) could evacuate all our patients.

We started loading up patients by priority and more staff from other floors brought up a few more Evac-Chairs and assisted us. It was all so chaotic.

Our stairwells have about 20 stairs, followed by a 'landing,' followed by about 10 more stairs.

Well, I was on the lower 10 steps, assisting one of the orderlies in transporting a patient, when I just happened to look up and see James at the top of the stairs. John was barely conscious, strapped to an Evac-Chair that James was piloting.

"What are you doing?" I exclaimed. "Don't do that!"

James was twitching when he said, "The man can't walk."

"You have to be trained to use this equipment," I sternly said to James. "Get someone to help you."

"But he can't walk," James repeated.

"I can't walk," John shouted with a slur. He then slumped forward and vomited on himself and down the first few steps.

James was so 'methed up' that he could barely walk. With John almost passed out in the chair, it was like the blind leading the blind.

I cursed under my breath. We had to get our patient out of the building, but I also had to try to convince the idiots at the top steps to stop what they were doing.

Before I could continue arguing with James and John, James tilted the chair back like you do when you're trying to get a stroller over a curb, and he took a step forward.

This is when crap got *really* crazy.

Gravity pulled John downward, and James couldn't keep a grip on the Evac-Chair, so the chair went tumbling down the stairs. John screamed as he bounced around, and his shrieks echoed throughout the stairwell. I couldn't let go of my Evac-Chair, or my patient would suffer the same fate.

"Go get help!" I ordered to James.

Did James listen? Of course not.

James tried to run down the steps to check on John, but he slipped on vomit and basically skated down the steps.

I don't know if it was nerves or what, but I started laughing and I couldn't stop.

"I'm okay," John said, face-down on the landing between the top and bottom portions of the stairwell, while still strapped in the Evac-Chair. "But I'm stuck."

I started laughing harder when James stood up and said, "Oh man, I have barf on my shoes."

Luckily, two staff members entered the stairwell to evacuate another patient, and they saw James and John. They called for help and we evacuated the rest of the floor.

What really made me angry was that five minutes later, the fire department gave the all-clear, and we had to transport all the patients back inside.

John and James were both arrested (they were both in possession of meth, shockingly), but first they had to go to the ER due to superficial injuries and complaints of pain that they sustained from their falls.

--O.R.
Indiana

<u>Idiots</u>

We received two males, both 25-35 years-old, via EMS for multiple injuries. One male, Mr. Smith, presented with a head injury and facial contusions. His friend, John, presented with dog bites to his calves, forearms, and hands. The patients were not critical, but their wounds were beyond the realm of superficial. John, we knew right away, would require surgery.

According to these men, their wives wanted to take a couple's shopping trip to a mall that was located three-hours away. The men did not want to go. They wanted to stay home and play video games. Their wives, however, did not wish to travel alone.

The men couldn't convince their wives to go without them, so Mr. Smith suggested the two men '*Bio-Dome* it.' None of us knew what that meant, until the men explained that there is in a scene in a movie, where two males attempt to get out of an outing with their girlfriends by injuring each other.

Apparently, while the men were at Mr. Smith's home, John hit Mr. Smith in the head with an iron fireplace poker. Mr. Smith fell face-first against his fireplace and became unconscious. He received four staples to close his head wound.

Mr. Smith's pit bull witnessed the attack from the back porch and jumped through a screen door to defend his owner. The dog attacked John, until John was able to lock himself in the bathroom and call 911. Mr. Smith regained consciousness prior to the arrival of EMS and crated his dog. The men then attempted to bandage their wounds with diapers.

When we brought up notifying the patients' wives, they both begged us not to. I don't know how they planned to explain their injuries to their wives. I can only imagine John being released from surgery to tell his wife something stupid and unbelievable like, "I fell."

Registration gets the props for convincing the men to notify their spouses.

I must say, the women took the news quite well for what had occurred, but they openly referred to their husbands as idiots. Mr. Smith's pregnant wife was most upset over the fact that the men had used diapers from her baby shower and left the nursery a disaster.

Mr. Smith was released with a script for pain meds, and John was transferred out. I guess they both got what they wanted, but there had to be a better way of getting out of a shopping trip.

--L.C.
South Dakota

Pain in the...

EMS transported a female in her late-teens to our ED. She had reportedly sustained a GSW, so our trauma team suited up, and we were ready. Officers were bringing in the shooter for medical clearance.

When the female arrived, she was lying on her side on the stretcher. She was screaming and crying all the way to her room.

Around the same time, two officers dragged in this kicking and screaming guy, who was probably in his early-twenties.

"Jane!" he called out. "Jane, where are you?"

"John!" she yelled from her room.

We had to restrain Jane with canvas straps because she kept trying to get up and get to the shooter's room. Officers handcuffed the shooter to his examination bed because he tried to do the same.

I entered the room with the doctor, and I started charting everything he observed. I looked down, and there was blood dripping down Jane's legs. I thought she'd maybe been shot in the thigh or something.

Close, but no cigar.

Jane was shot in cervix with a high-powered BB gun. The BB penetrated her cervix and was embedded. She required surgery to have the BB removed. I was really surprised at how much blood was present.

We had to go to John's room, too. He required sutures to a facial laceration that he sustained while fighting paramedics.

According to both patients, their idea of foreplay was John using his gun to pleasure Jane. He inserted the barrel of the gun into her vagina and accidentally fired a BB that was able to penetrate Jane's cervix because some kind of cartridge powered it.

Through all this, Jane seemed to be most upset that John was using a BB gun, not a 'real' gun. She seemed to like him for his 'bad boy' quality.

We tried to tell Jane that she was mighty lucky that John's gun wasn't a 'real' one, or she may have not lived through the ordeal.

John was arrested because he assaulted paramedics. He was also a felon with an open warrant, and he was in trouble for carrying a weapon.

--N.T.
Illinois

While at work, I used a pencil to scratch my inner ear. The hot pink, cupcake-shaped eraser top broke off, and when I tried to remove it, I pushed it further down the canal. I had to leave my shift early, register in the ER, and go under for a surgery that cost me $2,000 after insurance.

This is especially difficult to share because I am a 48-year-old male doctor and was on shift in the ER that night.

--N.P., M.D.
Wyoming

<u>Hysteria</u>

I recently discovered your books and am a little late to the party, but I wanted to tell a story that happened in the late-90s.

One night, when we were under a tornado warning, officers brought in one patient, while EMS brought us two. We didn't realize it at first, but all three patients were involved in the same altercation. The patient whom the officers transported had an ETOH level three times the legal limit, and he was medically cleared for skinned palms from a fall and minor contusions from fighting.

Our other patients, two middle-age females, were not so lucky. Jane's injuries included a fractured tibia, missing teeth, and a broken nose. Joan also sustained a broken nose, broken phalanges, and we discovered that she had a 3cm crack in her skull.

What's worse is that these women, apparently, hadn't finished their argument. Both left their beds and appeared to ignore their wounds as they threw punches at each other. Before we could break them up, they were on the nursing station's counter, beating the crap out of each other. Staff pulled the women apart and the officer on scene called for additional officers to monitor the women.

According to the police, Jane and the male patient went to confront Joan, who was the male's very-recent ex. The male not only demanded that Joan return his Pog collection, but he also claimed that since Joan was unemployed, her Beanie Babies collection belonged to him, citing he was the person who'd purchased the plush animals. Joan and Jane went at it, right after Joan hit her ex in the knee with a snow shovel. He attempted to break up the fight between his ex and new girlfriend, and he was injured in the process.

All these years later, I wonder if the three now feel foolish for fighting over toys that have depreciated with time?

--L.E.
Iowa

Uh, Hey...

During a mandatory training seminar, we noticed one of our new medics kept disappearing. He told our instructor that he was experiencing stomach discomfort, so we figured he had diarrhea. We started wondering if he had a condition he hadn't told us about, because he had disappeared on shifts, too. I guess we were just noticing the frequency of his absences because we were in a group.

Well, our instructor wanted to show us something that required boarding a rig and practicing on each other, so we headed to the nearest rig and opened the back doors.

The medic was standing in the back of the rig, with his BDUs and boxers around his ankles, and he was jerking off.

That's not even the craziest part of it.

This dude had a CVAD (Central Venous Access Device) hanging from his penis. He had inserted a tube into his penis.

When he realized he was busted, he quickly yanked the CVAD from his junk and ejaculated into a gauze pad.

Not only was this guy fired on the spot, but the police were also called, and he was arrested.

Annnnnd, *that's* not even the craziest part.

The guy admitted to doing this before and using the same tainted CVADs during patient care.

That's not the worst part, either.

He admitted to doing this while I was driving, while we were on the way to a call.

Seriously, I just thought he hated my music or something. I didn't know he was jerking off before we picked up a patient.

Awkward.

--Initials and location withheld at request

<u>Croak</u>

I had recently joined a home health organization that hired staff to sit with patients in their homes. My client's family hired me to stay overnight because he was 89-years-old and had a bad habit of sleepwalking.

The job was kind of boring, really, because while he was asleep in the other room, I just sat in the living room and watched TV or played games on my phone.

One night, I heard a loud noise from my client's bedroom, so I hurried to check on him.

My client's 22-pound cat had knocked a stack of library books off the dresser.

I picked up the cat and as I turned to leave, the patient broke wind. It was so loud that I probably would have heard it from the living room.

My patient sat up from a dead sleep, asked loudly, "Did y'all hear that bullfrog?", and then he laid back down and started snoring again.

I was laughing so hard that I accidentally dropped the cat, and I had to run out of the room because I was afraid I'd wake my client.

--S.W.
Kansas

<u>Unexpected Angel</u>

When I started as an ED nurse (back in the 70s), I was 22, newly-divorced from my abusive high school sweetheart (who moved us to a strange new city, beat me, and then filed for divorce so he could be with his mistress), had a toddler and one child on the way, and I was dirt poor. To make matters worse, my family lived across the country and I couldn't even save enough money to move back there.

One night, one of our frequents came in. We knew him quite well. He always came in for diabetic and COPD complications. He lived in a tiny camper he pulled behind this old rust-bucket and parked it wherever he could, for as long as he could. He wasn't particularly the best-dressed or cleanest patient. It was almost like he didn't care about his hygiene anymore. We'd all seen him around the city, where he'd be run off from businesses and residential areas for digging through dumpsters/trash cans. He bathed in the fountain at the park, usually at night. Every now and then, the hospital would allow him to use their facilities.

That night, I must admit, I was unnecessarily rude to Mr. Smith. I was rough when I was preparing him for a drip, and I cut him off when he tried to speak. I am still embarrassed over how I acted that night.

Mr. Smith didn't take any of my poor behavior personally, nor did he retaliate. This man could have very easily requested another nurse. He could have yelled at me or treated me how I was treating him.

"Honey," he said to me, "do you want to talk about it?"

"Talk about what?" I snapped. "There's nothing to talk about."

"I was married for thirty-seven years," he said with a smile. "I know how to tell when a woman's upset."

"You were married?" I skeptically asked. "You don't strike me as the marrying type."

Thankfully, he laughed off my rudeness once again and said, "I didn't always look this bad. When you lose someone as dear to you as my wife was to me, nothing else matters."

I nodded and remember turning away from him when tears started swelling in my eyes.

"I'm all-ears, if you want to get it all out," he offered.

I couldn't hold it in anymore. I explained to Mr. Smith all about my failed fairytale marriage, told him about how I was eating peanut butter sandwiches for breakfast, lunch, and dinner, how I could barely afford a sitter for my son, how I was so far from my family, and the most painful words of my life—right before I'd left for work that day, I'd received a phone call from my aunt; my mother had died, and I had no way to make it to her funeral. I told him that what I wanted most in the whole world was to just get back to my family, if only so my child(ren) could meet them.

I sat at the end of Mr. Smith's bed and I cried and cried and cried some more. He sat up and hugged me. A doctor heard me crying, saw me on the bed, and he sent me home for 'being too friendly' with a patient.

That night, my sitter told me she couldn't watch my son anymore because my check had bounced. I was in bad shape. My ex-husband basically took everything we had. I didn't know what I was going to do.

I fell asleep early and woke up with a major headache. As I was getting my son dressed, the phone rang. It was a fellow nurse.

"You need to get here as soon as you can," she told me.

"I don't have a sitter," I responded. I was afraid I was being called in for the incident that happened the night before. I thought they were going to fire me.

"No," the nurse said, "it's not bad. You're not going to believe this. Just come in, will you? Bring your kid with you."

I missed the bus and couldn't wait around for the next one, so seven-months-pregnant, I walked 14 blocks, pushing a stroller, to the ED.

The nurse hurriedly motioned for me to come over to her work area, and she held up a manila envelope.

"This is for you," she said. "That smelly guy came in a little bit ago and left it for you."

"What is it?" I asked.

She shrugged.

I cautiously opened the envelope and almost passed out.

Mr. Smith left an envelope filled with $4,500 for me. In 1974, that kind of money would be like someone coming to you today and giving you about $15,000, maybe even more.

With the cash, there was a short note scribbled on a napkin. It said to go back to my family and not to let a hard life break me.

At first, I only used enough money to pay a cab to drive me around to all the places I'd seen Mr. Smith. We finally found him at a park.

Mr. Smith refused to take the money back. He said I needed it more than he did, and he told me that he was much better off than everyone assumed he was. He told me that after his wife died, he wanted to live a 'simpler' life and that he didn't care about money or material things anymore. He said he was just basically waiting to die, so that he could be with his wife again.

I tried to keep in contact with Mr. Smith by writing letters to the hospital. He wrote a few back here and there.

Mr. Smith died a few years after he helped change my life. He donated enough to the hospital to have a hall named after him.

I left what little I had behind, and I moved back home. I named my second child after Mr. Smith (he got a tickle out of that). The money he gave me helped me buy a used car, find a place to live, and get myself back on my feet. I didn't have to worry about groceries anymore, and I was able to give my kids everything they needed.

I stayed in nursing and recently went PRN, just to stay active in my 'golden' years.

I don't know if Mr. Smith realized just how much he changed my life, but I will never forget him.

--M.K.

Then California, now Pennsylvania

We got wind of a frequent flyer going on the *Maury* show. You'd better believe that there will be a viewing party for that episode. Alcohol will be involved. We're already starting a pool for the first person brave enough to say something like, "You said this was the worst ER ever and that you were never coming back. Our lie detector determined…that was a lie."

--Anonymous at request

<u>Busted</u>

We were up to our eyeballs with patients, when something crazy happened.

I called the next patient and took him to the back. He had been begging for Oxycodone before we even made it to the treatment area, to cure his chief complaint: headache.

As soon as we walked by one of the rooms, a woman holding a towel to a cut on her arm bolted to the hallway and asked hysterically, "John, is something wrong with John Jr.?"

My patient stopped and replied to the female patient, "No. Why?"

"Uh, because you're at the hospital and you have him this weekend. If he's not hurt, where is he?"

I half-expected my patient to say the kid was in the waiting room with a friend, but he said, "At home."

"With who?" the woman asked.

My patient said, "Nobody. I'm not going to be here that long."

I knew for a fact, thanks to our computer system, that John had already been at the hospital for an hour.

"You left him alone?" the woman shrieked. "You left my son alone?"

"He doesn't need a damn babysitter every single time I go out," my patient said with a sigh.

"He is three years old!" the woman shouted.

The long-story-short is that the cops were called, and my patient was arrested.

He did *not* receive Oxycodone, either, but I bet he had a real headache when he was discharged in custody of law enforcement.

--T.L.

Georgia

Pick a Bone

I was working an ill coworker's overnight shift, and if it hadn't been for me filling in, I would have never believed her when she said night shifts are outrageous.

It was about 01:00 when a car screeched to a stop in front of the ER entrance. A woman hopped out from the driver's seat and ran inside as fast as her five-inch heels would allow.

"I need help," she shouted, panting. "Like, right now."

I picked up the phone to notify Charge that I needed assistance up front, and I asked the female, "Can you tell me what the injury is?"

"He's stuck. It's turning purple."

Hmmm.

Charge sent two RNs and one tech up to help our patient. They placed him in a wheelchair and rushed through the double doors to the back, all without saying a thing to me. They told the patient's girlfriend to register him at my desk.

It quickly became clear that this woman was not the patient's girlfriend. She stated she was his roommate's friend, who'd gone over to the patient's apartment and used her friend's extra key to wait at the apartment until her friend got off work. She couldn't tell me anything about the patient, other than his first name-which she couldn't even spell.

This woman told me that she heard the patient screaming and went to check on him, and that's when she knew they had to rush to the ER.

The patient, in his late-20s, had his penis stuck in what I think was a marrow bone. I don't exactly know what they're called, but I buy these for my dogs. They are thick, cylindrical bones that are usually filled with some sort of crunchy material. My dogs always eat the middles and carry the bones around for months.

I am not sure why this patient stuck his penis inside the bone, but nothing the nurses tried could get the bone to come off. I kept hearing that they needed to get the bone off immediately, or the patient could lose his appendage.

Charge called me and ordered me to call O.R. I had to page someone, just so we could get some kind of bone saw thing to the ER ASAP. The woman on the line gasped when I told her why we needed it.

It took a while, but the doctors freed the patient's penis from the bone. I don't think he suffered from any long-term damage.

That's the first and last time I worked a night shift. It was weird.

--N.I.
New York

She's Having a Baby

A few years ago, I transferred to this inner-city ER from a rural location, and it was a shock to my system, as at the rural ER, I very rarely was required to do much in form of actual security. At the new hospital, I found myself in a scuffle with a patient in the first 10 minutes on my first day. It became worse the longer I was employed there. It was more unusual to go home without bruises or soreness because we were battling patients and visitors hourly, it seemed.

At this place, we were also required to rotate positions. For example, two of us would be required to remain on OB, while one of us was required to be on each of the other floors. Two guards were stationed in the ER treatment area, and one guard was given a 'break' for the day (that's what management called it, but it was far from a break) by sitting at the ER registration desk. If the clerks had problems with patients, or if there was trouble in the waiting room, the guard in the ER registration area would be right there.

One day, this couple came in, and they acted like they were high. They were in their mid-late twenties and were chuckling. As soon as they'd stop, one would start up again, and then they'd both be laughing again.

Registration was getting pretty sick of waiting on them to tell them what they needed. They obviously couldn't have *that* much of an emergency if they could waste five minutes of everyone's time by just standing at the desk laughing.

"Can I help you?" the registration clerk asked for the millionth time. I could practically see the veins popping out of her temples.

"Yeah, we need to see if she's knocked up," said the male.

"You need a pregnancy test?" the clerk asked the girl.

"I just told you she did," the guy said.

They both giggled again, apparently proud of their rudeness.

"I have to speak to the patient," registration said. "Unless you're the one needing the test, I'm going to ask her the questions."

"What if she's a mute?" he laughed.

The registration clerk didn't skip a beat. She kind of bugged her eyes out, and right as I thought she was going to blow her top, she just kind of blurted out in a snap, "Then she can write it down."

The girl laughed, and the guy said, "Touché."

"Honey, I need your name, address, and phone number."

The male tried to speak for her, but registration cut him off abruptly and said, "What role do you play here?"

"I'm her boyfriend," he responded.

"I have to speak to *her* because *she* is the patient," registration repeated.

The girl giggled and gave her information to the clerk. She listed her boyfriend, John, as her emergency contact. They must have been on some good drugs, because they laughed nonstop.

While the girl was giving registration her information and signing consent forms, her boyfriend was wandering around the lobby, telling anyone he could see, "I'm going to be a dad."

Of course, when you hear someone say that, whether you mean it or not, you have a reaction to be nice and say, "Congratulations."

So, right there in the lobby, about 12 people told him congratulations, and they weren't even in the back to get the damn test yet. It was unbelievable.

The triage nurse came out of her office and called the girl back. Her boyfriend went with her. They were still laughing. Triage asked what was so funny, but the couple didn't respond; they laughed harder.

Since the triage room is so close to the registration area and is monitored for safety, we could hear everything. Triage tried to ask the girl questions, but her boyfriend continued to talk for her. It didn't seem like an abusive situation by any means, but it was just annoying.

"Will you let her talk for herself?" triage asked. "If you have a problem with this, feel free to remove yourself, because I can't give her a proper assessment. There are things that only she can answer."

"He can talk for me," the girl said with a cackle. "It's okay."

Triage had to wait about two minutes for the couple to stop laughing.

The nurse asked all the normal questions about medical history and stuff.

Triage asked, "Do you drink alcohol?"

The guy got all excited and said, "No way! You guys serve drinks here?"

"No," triage snapped. "I need to ask these questions for the triage process."

"Oh," he said, clearly disappointed. "Well, she doesn't like beer or wine, but she goes through a lot of vodka."

"Tobacco usage?"

"None of that. Just weed."

"Street drugs?"

The girl laughed and said, "If it's out there, I've tried it."

"If it's out there, she's on it," the registration clerk whispered to me.

I nodded. "Probably."

"And when was your last period?" triage asked.

"Well," John thought, "probably about three weeks ago, because that's when we do anal, so yeah, probably about three weeks ago."

Uhhh…

"Do you have a regular cycle? When would you expect your next period?"

The guy shrugged and said, "No clue."

Triage sighed.

"Next week, I think," the girl answered.

You've got to be kidding me.

"So, your cycle is not late or anything?" the nurse asked.

"No, but she needs a test."

"So," triage asked slowly, obviously irritated, "you decided to come to the emergency room, a week before your cycle is due to start, for a pregnancy test? Did you take one at home?"

"Hell no," the guy exclaimed. "Those things are, like, six dollars. Plus, they don't really work. Come on, everyone knows that."

He continued, "We went to the clinic, but they said they won't know till the end of the day."

"Hold up," triage said. "You two already went to a physician's office for this?"

"Yeah," the guy said. "Went to the clinic across town. They took her blood."

"For a pregnancy test, right?"

"Yeah."

"How long ago was this?"

"Maybe an hour."

"Twenty-five minutes," the girl spoke up.

The two started laughing again.

"But now you're in the emergency room…," triage said.

"Yeah."

Triage actually said, "Oh dear Lord," as she was walking the patients through the corridor to the treatment area. Registration and I were thinking the same thing.

Maybe five to ten minutes later, one of the guards in back radioed me and said he and the other guy were busy with a combative psychiatric patient. They wanted to know if I could come back and help one of the nurses with a problematic patient. I agreed, because even though I really didn't want to go, I couldn't say no and expect to keep my job.

When I went to the back, a nurse pulled me aside and told me John was harassing other patients, staff, and visitors.

I walked over to the room and saw John hanging out of the room. He was telling every person to pass by, "Hey, my girl's having a baby. I'm going to be a dad!"

"She hasn't even taken a test yet," a nurse in the room exclaimed.

"Sir," I said, "I need you to either stay in the room, or I need you to return to the waiting room."

"But I gotta tell everyone," he said.

"Well, you can tell everyone when your girlfriend is discharged," I replied. "I can't have you hanging out of the room. This is the emergency room, and we need to keep distractions to a minimum."

John said he would comply, so I went back to the front.

Maybe about 20 minutes later, John and his girlfriend left the ER. On the way out, he stopped everyone he saw and told them he was going to be a dad.

"I'm so glad they left," the triage nurse said, as she watched them walk out.

"New parents, huh?" I asked.

She took a sip of water and shook her head. "She's not pregnant. She's told us after the test that she's on birth control. Idiots."

Well, how about that.

--M.P.
Ohio

I once registered this guy for a finger injury. He and his girlfriend claimed it happened while he was using his fingers to pleasure her.

Yeah, he broke his finger.

If it happened the way they said it happened, I don't know if I should be impressed or if I should cringe.

--L.O.

Montana

Holy Matrimony

On my first night as a medic, my partner and I were dispatched to a hotel conference room for a report of an injured male with lacerations to his face. Dispatch said to also expect defensive wounds, and it was likely there would be multiple patients. An additional ambulance and officers were on the way.

When we arrived, the room was dark and there was still loud music playing. It wasn't difficult to figure out that this was a wedding reception.

In one corner, the groom was holding a towel to his face and had his head tilted back. There was cake on the floor, smashed into the carpet.

In another corner, about six people surrounded the bride. She was decked out like no tomorrow. Think of the biggest, fluffiest dress you could find, and then make it about three times bigger…and sparkly neon.

There were people fighting in the middle of the room. Wine and champagne glasses were broken all over the place. It was utter chaos. My partner said this was called a Romani wedding, or a 'gypsy' wedding.

We were first going to assess and treat the groom, but as we were crossing the room, this girl yanked the flag pole from the wall, and she hit another girl upside the head. That girl immediately fell unconscious, and therefore, became our priority. The girl who'd hit her tried coming after us, screaming, "Let her die!"

Another group of people dragged that girl off, and we assessed the unconscious patient.

By the time officers arrived, we were looking at five patients, and the bride was dangerously close to breaking away from her group to continue fighting.

We were trying to clean up the groom enough for transport, when the bride somehow got away from the police officers and came rushing over. She pushed me to the ground and started punching the groom in the head.

We gathered that, at some point during the reception, the bride 'discovered' the groom's ex on Facebook. The ex had pictures posted from her relationship with the groom, and the one that seemed to cause the issue here is a picture of the ex showing off her engagement ring…which was the same ring the groom gave to the bride.

"You couldn't even give me a new ring!" the bride shouted, as we tried to pull her away from the groom.

"It's a sodding heirloom," he shouted.

"You re-gifted my ring!" she yelled.

"It was my mother's ring," the groom shouted. "It was her mother's ring."

"But you gave it to Jane first! You couldn't be bothered to give me another ring!"

What a nightmare this was. It almost made me regret moving here, and I'm serious.

In the end, the bride was arrested, the groom received sutures, the flag pole girl was fine (but dizzy and sore), the girl who'd hit the unconscious girl was arrested, and various family members and friends were arrested as well, with charges that ranged from disorderly conduct to vandalism.

I have honestly never seen anything like this. My partner said this is more common than people believe, but I don't blame the culture, just the individuals involved.

--Initials and location withheld at request

Go Back to Class

One time, this college girl came to the registration window, and she appeared angry right out of the gate.

"Can I help you?" I asked.

"My roommate won't leave my stuff alone," she said.

"Uh, okay," I said.

"She keeps getting in my food, and she has sex on my bed when I'm in class, and now, I think she's using my stuff."

"Uh, this is the emergency room," I said. "Do you have a medical emergency?"

The girl nodded and started digging through this giant tote bag hanging from her shoulder.

I'm not even kidding…This girl pulled out two HUGE silicone vibrators from her bag, put them in the document slot under my window, and said, "I need you to test these and tell me if she's been using them when I'm not around."

I'm not afraid of sex or anything, and I'm not threatened by toys that are more endowed than I am, but I jumped back and screamed, "Oh, come on! Are you [effing] serious right now?"

One of the financial assistance clerks came out of her office to see if I needed her to call security.

"I don't know," I shouted, still worked up.

"But I didn't do anything wrong," the girl told the financial advisor and me. "She's the one using my stuff. Isn't that, like, illegal?"

The girl wouldn't accept my explanation that we couldn't test the sex toys for 'cross contamination,' so I had to go get a doctor. He laughed his butt off when she first explained what she wanted him to do, and then he just stared at her like she was dumb and said, "Oh my gosh. You're serious."

He then told the girl the same thing I did. He suggested that she lock up her belongings or file a request with her college administration office to find another roommate. She was yelling and cussing when she left, saying that we didn't know what we were talking about. She said she was going to sue the hospital and that she was going to post on Facebook that we refused to help her.

I don't know what happened with that girl because I never saw her again. I still can't believe she would just walk in a hospital and stick her fake, pink and purple penises through my window.

--N.H.
Florida

I once registered a patient whose chief complaint was that her dog licked his behind, and then gave her a 'kiss,' during which his tongue touched the inside of her mouth. She said she immediately drove to the ER and wanted to be tested for any disease(s) that her dog may have transferred to her via saliva.

--R.U.

Iowa

Hitchin' a Ride

The experience my partner and I shared resulted in a new company policy, and I still maintain it was no fault of our own.

We work in a rural setting, but we have more than enough runs to keep us busy. To save us some time and effort, the ER usually keeps the ambulance bay doors open, even after we pull in. We've never had to deal with anyone snooping around our vehicles while we've ben parked in the bay.

On the night in question, the ER was packed. We saw one of our frequents inside. I had wondered why we hadn't heard from him that night, but I guess it was because evening shift had already taken him to the hospital, where he'd been for hours. Now, he was getting on everyone's last nerve by begging for a ride to, well, anywhere. He refused to leave because it was raining, but the hospital staff didn't find his antics bad enough to call the police. Overall, he was just annoying.

Finally, a doctor handed this guy a twenty-dollar bill. He told the guy to call for a medi-cab, which is a rather pricey taxi system meant to be used for around-the-clock medical transport to and from the hospital. The guy disappeared, and I didn't think about him anymore.

We got all the signatures we needed and gave report of what we knew, and then we hung out with the nurses for a little while. Someone had brought in five-layer dip for a carry-in, and we hadn't eaten yet, so we considered it a fair break.

Dispatch called us and sent us packing to a fall. It was undetermined as to whether the call would be a transport or simple assessment and lift assist.

My partner and I took some dip for the road and drove out of town. I think the drive probably took about 10 to 15 minutes. The residence to which we were responding lived way out in the boonies, where there are no street lights or paved roads, so actually getting to the residence probably took another five minutes, once we were in the vicinity.

An elderly woman escorted us inside. She said her husband had tried to go downstairs for a drink, but he had missed a step and had fallen. He complained of minor leg and ankle pain. He did not think he needed medical transport, but his wife insisted, citing his recent cancer diagnosis.

Well, we were going to grab the stretcher, when we heard the patient's wife shriek from the living room. I went to see what was wrong, right around the time she was locking the dead bolt and scrambling to her phone.

"There's someone out there!" she panicked.

"Huh?" I asked. "Are you sure?"

She nodded and dialed 911. "I saw him. He was looking through my car window."

I looked at my watch. "It's three in the morning. Are you sure you saw someone? Do you think it could be a neighbor or something?"

"My nearest neighbor lives three miles that way," she pointed to the east. "And she's ninety. I doubt very much she's out for a stroll at this hour."

My partner and I decided that, hey, we were capable of handling an intruder/trespasser…hopefully, anyway.

I want to say that I fearlessly walked out the front door, but I was kind of scared. I watch a lot of scary movies and started thinking that I was going to end up butchered in the country.

We heard a noise and walked around to the side of the house.

There was our frequent—the same guy from the hospital—walking around this patient's yard.

"Uh, hey," he said to us. "Do you think I can get a ride back to town?"

Apparently, the guy didn't want to spend the cab fare the doctor had given him, so he thought he'd just hide in the back of our ambulance and 'hop off' at the next place we stopped. He didn't realize we'd be miles out of town.

We waited for an officer to arrive, and the frequent was arrested. During this time, our fall patient and his wife decided that they did not need medical transport after all, that they

316

would visit their primary physician if pain persisted the next day. They seemed more shaken of a trespasser than of the husband's fall.

Since that night, we are required to check the back before we start the engine. It's kind of annoying, and even though there's no real way to prove if we do it or not, I still check compulsively.

--W.J.
Nebraska

One time, we picked up this guy experiencing a bad LSD trip. He had to be restrained and eventually sedated because he was terrified of anything that was the color blue.

--C.H.

Washington

We had to call law enforcement for a combative overdose.

When officers arrived, one asked the man, "Where's your ankle bracelet?"

The patient responded that he removed the bracelet and attached it to his dog.

Our patient was arrested. And, since he violated his house arrest by trying to falsify his whereabouts, then went out and got high, he was sentenced to prison.

--K.L.
New York

Boom Goes the Boob

Me: 911, what's your emergency?

Caller: I need help.

Me: What's your emergency, ma'am?

Caller: I need an ambulance. I need to go to the ER.

Me: Can you tell me why? Are you injured?

Caller: Yes.

Me: Can you describe the nature of your injuries?

Caller: Yes.

Me, trying not to claw my eyes out: Please describe them.

Caller: My tit popped.

Me: It popped?

Caller: Yes.

Me: So, your breast implant ruptured?

Caller: Huh? No! I ain't got fake tits.

Me: No implants? You do have a breast injury?

Caller: Yeah.

Me: Can you elaborate on your injury?

Caller: What?

Me: How did it pop, ma'am?

Caller: I closed it in the door. I need help. My tit popped, and I don't want to die.

Me: I will notify EMS. Can you tell me if you're bleeding?

Caller: Yes.

Me: Are you able to control the bleeding?

Caller: I'm not bleeding.

Me: You're not bleeding?

Caller: No, I just popped my tit. How long before someone gets here?

Me: Someone will arrive shortly.

Caller: I have to call my boyfriend. He's going to be pissed.

The caller was on a meth high and was arrested for possession and attempting to distribute meth while she was admitted to the emergency room. Yes, genius tried to sell meth to nurses.

And no, she didn't 'pop' her tit. It was just bruised, according to our medics.

--H.B.
Indiana

<u>When it Rains...</u>

I was training a new girl, when one of the nurses told me there was pizza in the lounge. I asked the new girl if she felt she could hold down the fort for a few minutes, while I heated up a few slices and grabbed a drink. She was trained enough to register a patient, but she was still having trouble taking admit calls and transferring patients in the computer. She said she would hold any calls or requests like that until I got back, if she received them.

I had just finished heating up my pizza and was trying to juggle the plate, along with a tiny Styrofoam cup filled to the brim with soda. All the sudden, the new girl came running around the corner. She ran right into me, and I spilled pizza and soda all over myself and the floor.

"He has a gun!" she screamed. "He has a gun!"

Screaming this in an ED where we do not have security left everyone scrambling to hide. I didn't know where else to go, so I hid inside this metal warmer where we keep sterilized blankets. I could hear nurses and patients screaming, and someone yelled out that they were on the phone with 911.

I felt like I was going to die in the blanket warmer. It really wasn't as hot as you'd think it would be, but I was scared. I was drenched in sweat, soda, and had clumps of cheese and pepperoni stuck to this $60 white shirt I'd just bought that morning. I had to pee, and I felt like I couldn't breathe.

A few minutes later, I heard officers yelling, and then I heard an officer come to the ED and tell everyone they could come out, that the situation had been resolved and we were safe.

I came out of the blanket warmer and my coworker was leaning against the counter, laughing hysterically.

"It was an umbrella," she choked. "They said it was just an umbrella."

"Wait," a doctor sternly said. "Are you telling me you had everyone panicking and fearing for their lives because someone came in with an umbrella?"

She shrugged and said, "I thought it was a gun."

I think we were all grateful that she alerted us of a possible shooter, but we were all kind of mad that she caused the panic in the first place.

I'm glad I'm still alive, but I couldn't save that $60 shirt. I'm still kind of pissed about it because the new girl didn't show up for work the next day. She said the ED was boring, so she just decided that a no call-no show was the best way to quit her job.

--D.W.
Delaware

He Tried

I work in a rural ED and admit that I cannot relate to stories of gore and trauma. Most of our patients are in-and-out, with exception to patients presenting with CVA markers or coronary complications. In a year, I think we've seen (in our ED, not only on my shift) three to five 'traumas.' Two of those patients were from the same MVA and were life-lined out because our facility cannot support much more than sutures. In a sense, we are what most of us call a 'nurse's hut.' Medics call us the 'Band-Aid Box.'

Well, a few years ago I was working the evening shift, when EMS called report to 'get the copter in the air right now.' We trust our medics, so we called for a flight to be dispatched to our ED. EMS told us to 'get all the doctors possible.' It sounded pretty scary! I was running my butt off, trying to find everything the team needed and check the crash cart, so I didn't know what to expect.

When I saw medics rolling the stretcher down the hall, I thought I was going to pass out. I'd never seen anything like it in my life, and I didn't know how the patient was still alive.

This man, in his mid-to-late 30s, was lying on his side with a 15" lawn mower blade impaled from his lower back to his abdomen. We were sure the blade pierced the man's organs.

Believe it or not, he was relatively calm, though there were times he strained to remain conscious before his pain meds kicked in and knocked him out.

This man told his nurse something about 'National Light Night' or some event taking place around the globe, where people were encouraged to turn off their lights for an hour. It was supposed to make a visible impact and argument for global warming.

The patient, a farmer who does side work as a blade sharpener, was in his basement, searching for a battery-powered lantern *after* he had cut power to his electricity. I don't know if he wasn't thinking or what, but he climbed on his work table and reached for the shelf above it. He then lost his footing and landed on a blade that he still had positioned in his sharpener clamps.

Luckily, the patient's wife heard the commotion, turned the electricity on, and called 911.

I don't know too much about the patient's injuries, other than the blade did go through and through his gallbladder. He was life-lined to a trauma facility, loaded up on lots of good drugs to keep him comfortable.

--Y.W.
Oklahoma

__Boyfriend Material__

We have to ask patients their occupations. One man told me his occupation was a meth dealer. At first, I didn't know if he was serious. Then, he pulled out a case filled with syringes that were filled with drugs. He acted like I should've been impressed, and he started hitting on me! He kept saying things like, "I can provide," and, "You want some, baby? I got you."

I notified the patient's nurse, doctor, and our ES supervisor. They all told me to call the police.

I felt really bad about it, but I did call the police.

They came and arrested the patient, who'd only registered because he thought he'd caught strep throat.

--Initials and location withheld at request

Sad

EMS called in a drowning, and since it was 03:00 on a weekday, we wondered how it was possible. When we received the patient's stats and personal details, we were even more shocked and confused.

Our patient was in her 90s. She was a frail thing, weighing no more than ninety-pounds. It was frightening to see EMS performing chest compressions because it looked like they were going to break this poor woman in half. In our ER, our physician performed an emergency tracheostomy and pulmonary toilet.

Unfortunately, though our patient showed vague signs of life, she could not thrive without artificial ventilation and life support.

The patient's caretakers avoided many of our questions and it was obvious that they were lying, when they did answer questions. They told us many versions of what had occurred, but finally seemed to settle on the story that they had been sleeping, when they heard a noise and found our patient face-down in the bathtub. Our patient was dressed in a nightgown upon arrival, and we noted contusions to her neck and shoulders, as if someone had applied force to these regions. She also presented with bruising consistent with wrist restraints.

Law enforcement was notified, and officers questioned the families and called out the variations in their stories. For three people claiming they were fast asleep and woken by their relative's noise, they sure changed their stories a lot, and nothing was adding up.

One by one, the family members started confessing.

Apparently, the patient had been displaying 'bizarre' and violent behavior. The family, instead of seeking medical attention, began seeking answers in faith. They believed the patient was possessed by a demon or Satan.

The patient's family kept her restrained and bedridden. They admitted to starving her for days, hoping to 'run out' the 'evil spirit' living inside of her. They allowed her to stew in her own excrement.

Finally, the family decided to attempt an exorcism. They filled the bathtub with water, ice, and 'holy oils' they had ordered through a mail-order catalogue. They then submerged the patient in the water and held her until she stopped thrashing. They admitted to holding her under the water for an additional two minutes.

Unfortunately, this patient passed away due to this family's medical neglect. She was determined to have a UTI, which often presents as Altered LOC in elderly patients. Any healthcare professional will be able to suggest testing for UTI in elderly patients presenting with 'off the wall' behavior, and this can often be treated in virtually no time, after treatment has begun and meds have been calibrated.

I cannot tell you what happened to the patient's family, other than they were arrested that night. This story has haunted me ever since, though it has been many years since it occurred.

I urge all families with elderly relatives, if you notice that your family member is behaving strangely, whether violently or just acting 'weird,' please reach out to medical professionals to help. Please do not attempt to take matters into your own hands or administer holistic medications until you have a proper diagnosis. I think it goes without saying that I would also never recommend an exorcism or the abuse this patient endured in her final days.

--Initials and location withheld at request

<u>Gag</u>

The weirdest/grossest thing I've ever registered a patient for was a complaint of "I lost my credit card."

The 450-pound patient stated she routinely placed her debit card in her vagina overnight, due to her adult son 'robbing [her] blind' while she slept. Instead of, I don't know, buying a safe, she stored her cards and wads of cash in her cooter.

Her nurse told me that they were in the middle of the exam, when the patient stated she had forgotten that she'd used her card that morning and had stashed it in her bra!

The worst part about all of it was when it was over. The woman had to come to my desk to pay her co-pay. She tried to hand me her card, and then acted like I was the worst person in the world because I put gloves on first.

After she left, I made everyone wait in line while I used Sani-wipes on everything in my workspace.

--I.K.
Georgia

Fourscore and Seven Years Ago

Our patient was transported to us via EMS, badly beat to a pulp. Using only Spanish, he hysterically screamed that Abraham Lincoln had beaten him up. It reminded me of an episode of *Supernatural,* when Abe Lincoln's wax statue killed a character, so I couldn't stop wondering what the patient had experienced. Whatever the case, the patient was so hysterical that he had to be sedated. He required surgery for his injuries.

We all thought the man was crazy, right, until officers brought in a man for a med-clearance.

Yep, this dude was dressed like Abraham Lincoln, from a fake beard to the stovepipe hat. Apparently, he was dressed that way because he was working as one of those sidewalk sign-slingers at a quick-loan place. He just up-and-decided that he'd make more money by mugging people on the streets.

The po-po took Abe Lincoln to jail that day, and we had to call downstairs to surgery to tell the nurses what happened. They said the patient was still freaking out when he was finished in surgery, so they explained the situation and the patient calmed down.

--E.M.
California

Remodel

My husband and I had just gotten our tax refund, and my goal was to completely redecorate the house. My husband complained that I never let him help, so I assigned him the task of redecorating the master bathroom.

Honestly, he did a great job. He chose a beautiful white shower curtain that had silver roses and leaves printed on it, purchased the nicest bath towels I've ever seen, and he found a white mat set. I was quite impressed.

He kept hounding me to take a shower, so I thought maybe I worked up a stinky sweat—that, or he was going to try to sneak in the shower with me. I showered like usual, though.

When I stepped out of the shower, I panicked. There was blood on the shower mat when I pressed my foot down, and I was dripping blood on the mat. I couldn't have cut myself because I didn't feel it. I started thinking I was experiencing vaginal bleeding and panicked because of health complications in my family line.

I was so freaked out by all the blood that I fell forward and stabbed myself in the forehead on the towel rack. There was blood everywhere.

I staggered out to the bedroom, where my husband was lying on the bed, watching television. I didn't even have a towel on, but I had my hand pressed against my wound and told him I needed help.

He jumped from the bed, tripped on the cat, and sliced his ear on a cedar chest we keep at the foot of the bed.

Neither of us could drive, so we had to call my daughter to take us to the ER. Between the two of us, we received 16 sutures.

I learned that the bath mat my husband had purchased was a Halloween decoration! It was *supposed* to look like blood when it was wet. My daughter found the whole thing hilarious because she's the one who convinced my husband to do it in the first place. She was behind his pleas to be in charge of decorating the bathroom; he confessed that he didn't care if the bathroom was blue or painted like rainbows, that it was 'just a good place to take a crap and brush [his] teeth.'

I was frustrated with my daughter for a while, but it was short-lived.

--D.Z.
Nevada

We had a prostitute come in one night, claiming her John had 'effed her too hard.' She said he never choked, hit, or abused her during their session, but she wanted us to document that he did not 'make love gently,' because he was a well-known attorney and she thought she would be able to extort money from him.

Yikes.

--M.E.
New Jersey

Stay Off the Internet!

We are all well aware of the 'Web M.D. Syndrome,' a 'condition' that strikes us when we're searching for answers online. You type in that you have a headache and runny nose, and all the sudden you read that you could be dying of an infection that you caught from some stranger at the store who was in contact with spotted frogs from Central Asia. Hey, paranoia happens to the best of us.

Here are a few crazy chief complaints sent in by ER workers, taken from patients presenting after surfing the web:

My 19-year-old patient said he was watching porn, when he started thinking that something was wrong with his penis. He was worried because he wasn't as 'big' as the guy in the X-rated flick. Our doctor told the kid that it was just a sad part of life.

--A.H.

A couple brought their kid in at 02:00 for an odd string of complaints. According to the parents, they were concerned because the child couldn't walk without falling, still wasn't potty-trained, and the child couldn't identify common household items. They went online and were convinced the kid had a neurological disorder. They demanded scans and tests.

Our doc explained to the couple that the child was ONE, and that all this behavior was normal.

--K.S.

Arkansas

We once had a 42-year-old divorcee come in and request the 'virgin surgery' that she read about on some crackpot website. She was convinced that, if she had this surgery, she'd be able to get any man she wanted because 'all men want virgins.'

I don't know how she planned to explain her four kids, all of whom she brought along with her to the ER and made sit in the room while we explained why we couldn't do this.

--T.G.
North Carolina

New parents complained that their newborn was 'crying all the time,' so they were worried that she had an undiagnosed disorder. They went to a website and printed five pages of things that could be wrong with the baby, and they wanted us to check for all of them.

They hadn't fed the baby in six hours, and the child had a diaper rash.

We had no choice but to turn them over to Family Services, after one of them mentioned taking illegal drugs.

--F.T.
Texas

"So, this *Buzzfeed* quiz said I might be a sociopath. I need someone to tell me I'm not, because I'm supposed to get married in three days."

--R.Y.
Colorado

"My mom just posted on Facebook that my cousin has Syphilis, and I need to be checked."

We thought the patient was just stupid, but he tested positive and admitted to having sex with his first cousin.

Awkward.

--Initials and location withheld at request

Patient: "This thing said coffee enemas help you lose weight."

Me, Triage: "Uh, okay?"

Patient: "I'm wearing one of my grandpa's diapers."

Me: "Uh…"

Patient: "I can't stop pooping, and it's bad. Like, it's real bad. It's not solid *at all*. I don't know what I did wrong. I used coffee from Starbucks."

Me: "Uh…"

--M.M.
Maine

A 16-year-old male attempted to register in our ES for priapism (a painful erection that will not go away). He told us that he read on the internet that it was possible to get high by consuming an unspecified dosage of Viagra that had been crushed up and mixed with at least eight ounces of prune juice. He said he crushed up two of his dad's pills and used prune juice he'd purchased at the store. According to the boy, the contents of the Viagra and prune juice were supposed to create a chemical reaction that resulted in 'tripping.'

The patient then told us that he'd spent the last six hours with diarrhea and a painful erection. He drove his parents' car to the ES and told us he wanted to be released before a certain time, because his parents were on their way home from a weekend trip out of town.

Unfortunately, our policies prohibit registering a minor without parental/guardian consent, so we couldn't do anything until we contacted the boy's parents. The kid was so upset that he had a panic attack and collapsed on the lobby floor after holding his breath.

The kid's parents gave us verbal consent to treat their son, and they arrived about an hour, hour and a half after we called them.

We thought the patient's mother was going to have a stroke as she was yelling at him, but the kid's dad thought it was hilarious.

The most memorable words from the father to his son were, "Being stupid hurts, doesn't it?"

Helping Hands

Jane, 82 and recently widowed, called 911 one night, to report that her light bulb went out, and she couldn't reach to change it.

Our dispatcher was a jerk to Jane and scolded her on abusing emergency services. Dispatch told Jane not to call back, or law enforcement would be sent to Jane's house and she'd be fined or arrested for calling 911 for non-emergencies.

When the dispatcher went around *bragging* about it, we managed to find the identifying information from call records, and two of us went over to Jane's house, completely unexpected.

Jane's kitchen ceilings were about 12-feet high. She'd been cooking by candlelight for three days before we arrived. She was in tears as she explained that she was afraid all the lights were going to burn out, eventually leaving her to live in the dark. Her husband had been in charge of changing light bulbs, and Jane had no family to help her anymore.

Jane wanted to pay us for our services, but we refused. She insisted that we take butterscotch candies.

We each gave Jane our personal phone numbers and told her to give us a call if she ever needed help.

Our dispatcher wasn't written up because our boss said she was *technically* correct on how she handled the call, but she was warned not to be such a coldhearted bitch to the elderly.

--J.W.
Kansas

Surprise!

We were packed one night, so we were pulling select patients to the side of the waiting room to monitor temps and the like. Patients with severe fluctuations would be called back sooner, and the rest would have to keep waiting.

I went to the waiting room and called a patient to check her blood pressure. She was wearing a long, wool pea coat, black leggings, and cowboy boots.

"Ma'am," I said, "I'm going to check your blood pressure. Can you remove your coat for me?"

She took off her coat and was topless! She didn't seem to think it was at-all strange that she had her breasts out for the entire waiting room to see. Even as I scrambled to hand her coat back to her and cover her up with my arms, she just kind of looked at me like I was crazy and that it was completely normal to be half-naked in front of 50 people.

I rushed her to a consult room, where she continued to wait because we had no additional beds open. I didn't think it would be right to leave her in the waiting room after that.

--A.W.
Ohio

<u>Yum</u>

One of my patients came to my office with a walk-in complaint of 'body odor.'

It did not take long to pinpoint the source of said odor.

The patient, a 20-something female who was gung-ho about saving the environment, made what she called a 'junk glob' of 'deodorant' that you and I would immediately toss in the trash can, just by its curdled, brown appearance.

This 'junk glob' consisted of bacon grease, oregano, rose-scented bath oils, Vicks Vapor Rub, and I can't even remember the rest of the ingredients. Yes, the smell masked her natural odor, but I would have rather smelled her sweaty armpits than have been subjected to even ten seconds of what she'd been using. It made me think of a story about a dentist in one of your books.

All I know is this woman stunk to high Heaven, and I had to ask my cleaning service to air out my office overnight, even though we tossed the 'junk glob' in the trash and took the trash out almost immediately.

I worked with the patient to find an all-natural replacement and recommended to her a few organic and holistic shops around the city. I made her promise that she would never make any hygienic items from internet recipes unless she consulted a professional first.

--J.Y., M.D.
Alabama

Extra Help

On overnight shift, as you know, it is difficult to manage when you are shorthanded in the emergency room. This was the case for our shift. We were down three nurses, had no techs, and our orderly was sent home after vomiting *on* a patient. Influenza hit our department, and it hit us hard.

Especially because it was the middle of the night, we were having a heck of a time finding people to come in. Only one day-shifter would commit to coming in early, but he said the earliest he would be able to make it would be an hour before his shift normally began. It wasn't a help at 02:00, but it was a little bit of help, and we would take anything we could get.

Oh, it was a nightmare. Our unit clerk was working as fast as she could. Tensions were high, and this poor woman was getting the brunt of all of our frustrations. Our doc was shouting orders at her left and right, and we weren't much different. On top of that, the

355

unit clerk was responsible for cleaning rooms. We were packed. On a normal night, we see about 20 patients. On this night, just three hours in, we'd already seen 54 patients. That was just the beginning. The waiting room was so full that people were sitting on the floor and in the hallways. Security was out in full-force for patients angry about the wait times. We had addicts going through withdrawal in the lobby, and at the same time, we had patients tweaking in the waiting room. We had MVAs pouring in like you wouldn't believe, and I think we were all waiting for a meteor to crash down and take the pain away. Our Nursing Supervisor pulled all available staff from other floors, but other departments were just as busy as we were, so we lucked out by getting one nurse. One.

Fast forward to about 03:00, when EMS transported a LOL to us from her SNF. Her chief complaint was Alt LOC, joint stiffness, fever, loss of appetite, and depression. She was 91-years-old.

When this patient first arrived, we didn't have an open bed. We had to leave her in the hall, still loaded to the EMS stretcher, and we assessed her in the hall.

The patient seemed 'zoned out.' She barely responded to us, but she did tell us she was not experiencing pain and that she was 'just tired.' She asked for a blanket, and then she told us that she wanted to be left alone. We assured her we would get her in a room and begin proper treatment as soon as we had a room available.

"As you can see," the doctor said, "we are in a bit over our heads with sick patients tonight."

She said, "It's okay, dear. I was a nurse for forty-six years. You take your time."

Halleluiah! Finally, a patient who understood that we were all one person with two hands and two legs!

About 20 minutes passed, and EMS called in SIX MVA patients en route. Due to the circumstances of their accidents, they were all considered traumas. Medics stated most of the patients appeared fine, except for complaints of pain and some minor lacerations. Two, however, were in bad shape.

When the patients arrived, we still didn't have beds. Charge was pissed and took it out on everyone in the room. The unit clerk finally lost her mind. She stood up, threw a stack of papers to the floor, and shouted, "I am only one damn person! I can't do everything. How hard is it for one of YOU to get room eight a blanket? It would take two seconds for someone sitting right next to the coffee pot to give five's husband a cup. I can't do everything for you!"

Our Nursing Supervisor took her aside and did breathing exercises with her. The unit clerk returned to her area, picked her papers up off the floor, and was crying as she was trying to reorganize all the papers. Charge called over to Pediatrics and begged to use any open beds. They accepted, so we started moving some of our lesser-symptomatic/ill patients over that way.

Someone told me to take our LOL over to Peds, so I went to her stretcher, but the stretcher was empty.

"Where's my lady?" I yelled.

There was so much commotion that nobody had heard me.

"Hello?" I screamed. "My patient has disappeared."

"Probably a walk-out tired of waiting," someone blindly suggested. "Good riddance. If you can't stay for treatment, it wasn't an emergency in the first place."

"My patient was secured to a stretcher and is ninety-one," I shouted with a grunt. "She didn't just get up and walk out."

Of course, nobody had seen anything. I was close to tears. Call lights were going off every-which-way, patients were screaming (both in pain and just to be jerks because they were tired of waiting), the place was a mess, and though it felt like two hours had passed, only a few minutes had gone by.

EMS crashed through the doors and yelled, "Here's your code!"

Code? Code? What code? Oh, that's right, the code that was called in when the unit clerk was having her meltdown. It was the code our doc took but forgot to tell anyone about.

As I was assisting with the code, I just happened to lift my head at just the right moment to see my LOL by the coffee pot. She was juggling a stack of blankets in the crook of her elbow, had a pillow pinched between her fingers, and was carefully carrying a cup of coffee in her left hand.

All I could remember thinking is, 'What in the world is she doing?'

Our OD code expired, so I left the room and was on a mission to track down my LOL. I searched everywhere, and I mean everywhere. I couldn't hold my bladder anymore, so I headed to the back to use the employee restroom.

There was my LOL, walking away from our open supply closet, her arms full of cleaning supplies and trash bags.

"Room seven will be ready in just a minute," she said with a sweet smile. "I just finished four and twelve. Nine's wife will need more tea shortly. She's a nervous Nelly, don't you know?"

I didn't know what to say, and I didn't have time anyway, because my LOL went powerwalking away like she was on a mission, with her pink house shoes shuffling on the tile, and the mid-strap on her blue bath robe dragging behind her.

I'm not going to lie, first things first: I went to the bathroom.

My LOL had room seven cleaned by the time I finished, washed up, and was ordered to discharge a patient. She was the quickest room-cleaner we had, and she wasn't even on our staff.

Of course, we had to tell Mrs. Smith to stop, and she had a fit about that. She said that, as a nurse, it was her job to recognize when help was needed, and "Sweetie, y'all need help."

She seemed to understand when I explained that we couldn't allow her to wander freely, due to liability for her and because she was violating HIPAA by wandering to patient care zones, but that didn't mean she was any less angry with us for telling her to stay in her room…the room that we finally got her into because SHE cleaned it.

Mrs. Smith was treated for a UTI and another minor non-communicable ailment, before we discharged her back to her SNF. She seemed bitter that we wouldn't allow her to help out more.

Honestly, during the time she was working her butt off, our department *did* run a lot smoother than it had before she arrived. And, as soon as we took her off the floor, things went right back to being chaotic. Maybe we should have made her an honorary staff member that night.

--T.R.
Louisiana

My patient registered at 04:00 with the chief complaint, "My husband passed out."

Did my patient pass out?

No.

She wanted to be seen to 'make sure' she didn't have what he had.

He had low blood sugar.

The husband (brought in by EMS) was livid when he found out his wife registered, too.

--A.Y.

South Dakota

Food for Thought

I work as a receptionist for O.R., and I could tell you a million stories. I'll settle for this one, because it blew my mind. Common sense is clearly not common.

Me, at 04:00, before having my coffee: Good morning.

Woman, slurping from a fast food soft drink and cramming a hash brown in her mouth: Hi. They told us to check in here.

Me, looking to the woman's husband: Ah, having a surgery this morning? Most people come in, looking nervous. You seem very relaxed.

Husband: *Laughs* Oh, I'm not the one having the surgery. My wife is.

Me: Ma'am, are you scheduled for surgery this morning?

Woman, still slurping on her drink: Yeah.

Me: Did the nurses and doctors not tell you about the food policy?

Husband: But they said don't eat at home.

Woman: Yeah, they didn't say anything about eating here or in the car.

Me: Uh...

Woman: *Accidentally spits part of a breakfast sandwich on me as she's speaking with a full mouth* They only tell people that because most people eat such unhealthy food, anyway. If you go out to eat, you're getting better than what you'd make for yourself.

Me: Uh, no. There are legitimate medical concerns about eating prior to a surgery.

Husband: *Laughs* No, there are not.

Me: I'm sorry, but I'll have to notify the doctor. It's very unlikely he will want to risk the surgery, knowing you are eating less than an hour before you're supposed to go under anesthesia.

I notified the doctor and he denied the surgery, which was really no surprise. The patient and her husband became irate, and the patient threw her half-full cup of orange soda at me. We called security and the two were escorted from hospital property. Another hospital called a few weeks later, requesting the patient's medical records. I guess she decided to have her surgery elsewhere.

--E.G.
Utah

I registered a patient for 'penis pain' at 06:00.

Turns out, the man had a true emergency.

He was transferred to surgery stat because he stuck a pencil up his wee-wee. It was apparently all the way in there, as in the nurses couldn't visibly tell there was a pencil in there, besides some swelling and redness.

His nurse said he told her that he just wanted to see what it felt like.

Who sticks a pencil in his wee-wee at six in the morning?!

--L.H.
Virginia

You Got Some 'Splainin' To Do

I work in Pediatrics, and our unit depends on donations from the community and our staff to stock the waiting room with things to keep kids busy. Unfortunately, most of our toys are geared for younger children, so we have the 'go-to' toy that you see in *every* doctor's office *ever*: that wire thing with wooden balls that slide. We also have a table that's painted to look like a road, with wooden cars that are missing wheels and barely resemble cars anymore. The toys are mostly for children between the ages of 2 and 4, which leaves the older kids bored to tears…which results in them running wild and barreling through our waiting area like F-5 tornadoes. This isn't particularly enjoyable for our parents or our staff. The last thing anyone wants to deal with while a child is admitted to the hospital is having to discipline their other children.

Well, I took monetary donations and decided I would go to our local thrift shop to see what I could find for our older kids.

I found some dolls, coloring books, and old *Highlights for Kids* magazines. Those things were a start.

I was just about to leave, when I saw a bundle of graphic novels (like comics), all stacked together and secured with rubber bands. We'd been seeing an influx of siblings ranged 12-15 in our waiting rooms, and I know my own kid *loves* to read those things, so I checked the price with the clerk. One-dollar for a stack of 12 graphic novels was a steal.

When I got to work that day, I unloaded the loot in the waiting area. I removed the rubber bands from the stack of comics and kind of tossed them on the table. The teens and pre-teens in the waiting room snatched them up like I had tossed out money. Even a few younger kids were grabbing them. Man, I was so proud of myself for thinking to buy those.

Not even fifteen minutes later, while I was clarifying a med-order with a patient's doctor, an elderly woman I identified as a patient's grandmother, came marching to my work station and shouted, "I want to know who put those magazines in the waiting room."

I placed the doctor on hold and asked, "The comic books?"

"Yes!"

"I did," I beamed. "The store had them at such a great price that I just couldn't pass them up. I thought the kids would love them."

"What is wrong with you? Why would you let any kid read this filth?"

"Huh?" I asked. "I let my son read them, and he loves them, too."

The woman scoffed and snapped, "You are a horrible mother, and you're a horrible nurse. You have no business working with children."

I was so confused, so I told the doctor I would call him right back, and I went to the waiting room.

The old woman kept slapping her grandson's hands as he kept reaching for the comics on the table.

"Disgusting," the woman muttered. "That's what this place is."

I picked up one of the comics and started flipping through it. It didn't take long to realize why the old woman was so angry.

These comics were not meant for children. I think that was evident, especially by the animations of characters having sex. There was one very graphic oral sex scene. The language matched the pictures.

Every-single-one that I picked up and flipped through was like that!

I looked over and saw two teenage boys each reading a comic. They both had grins that stretched from ear to ear.

I hurried over and snatched the comics from each boy. My face was as red as an apple. I have never felt more embarrassed or ashamed in my life!

I tried to explain to the old woman what happened, but she wasn't hearing it. Instead, she reported our unit to H.R. I had to write a report stating that I had accidentally purchased and placed cartoon pornography in our waiting room. The H.R. head understood the complaint, but he found the situation hilarious and just gave me a warning to pay more attention if I made future purchases.

I am grateful that I did not get written up, but I still feel embarrassed that I allowed that woman's six-year-old to see that type of material.

--J.N.
California

Glorified Customer Service

Healthcare professionals chime in with real comments left on Press Gainey patient satisfaction surveys. I don't miss dealing with people like this! Good grief!

"I signed in for a sore throat. They took this guy back, just because someone shot him. We all have problems. He needed to wait his turn."

--L.K.
Illinois

"By the time the girl brought me the coffee I asked for, it was cold. She said she was part of a code. Totally unacceptable."

--E.H.

"I set my alarm for my meds. The nurse said it was PRN, not when my alarm went off. My Medicaid is paying her salary. You need to tell your nurses that they have to do what patients say."

--M.M.
Florida

"I had to listen to this woman crying for an hour. I don't care if her husband died or not, I was trying to watch the news."

--N.L.
West Virginia

"They told me not to put that inside me again. What I do in my own bedroom is none of their business."

We know this came from a patient who'd registered for a vintage soda bottle inserted in his rectum. It was made of glass and suctioned itself in his rectum. It took us thirty minutes to remove the bottle, and the patient was crying the entire time.

--M.J.
South Carolina

"The [string of expletives] nurses said I fit drug-seeking behavior. Obviously not, because I came to the ER instead of going to a dealer."

--H.I.
New Jersey

"The beds at [next county's hospital] are much softer. I'll be going there next time. Get new beds!"

--T.R.
Texas

"If I have to sit in the waiting room for two hours because your staff can't grasp time management, the least you could do is order the sports package [from the cable company]."

--B.H.
Kansas

"They made me drink something for heartburn. It was disgusting! I can't believe you can get away with torturing patients. Just because you're doctors, doesn't mean you can make people take medicine like that. Something must be wrong with you to make it taste that way."

I remember this patient. She seemed to think we had a flavor bar down at pharmacy. She also sued the hospital because she was allergic to her gown's material and was angry because we didn't have gowns she *wasn't* allergic to. She lost.

--L.M.
Indiana

"I'm telling all my friends not to come here or bring their pets here. If I was too scared to off myself, I'd come back and let one of your nurses do it for me, like they killed my husband."

Firstly, this lady's husband died two *months* after he was admitted to our hospital, and the coroner said he died from a heart attack. Secondly, we'd prefer that you don't bring your pets to an emergency room; take them to the vet like everyone else. And third, we didn't get this review until *after* the patient was denied Percocet for 'hair pain.'

Remind me, please, why did I think nursing was going to be a great career?

--S.R.
New York

"How am I supposed to get any sleep when they keep coming in and asking me to rate my pain? Then, they told me I can't stay the night? They kicked me out. I told them my girlfriend kicked me out, but they made me leave, anyway."

--A.R.

Washington

"I've had better coffee from a run-down Super 8. Ridiculous."

--D.W.

Florida

You never know if you're going to be a fight or flight during an emergency.

What will I do if a patient falls out of a wheelchair in front of me?

Apparently yell, "Oh shit!"

--*Anonymous*

Invention of the Century

My partner's sister had an emergency and he was the only one 'available' to watch her 2-year-old son, even though he was on duty.

A bunch of us gave the kid chocolate, gave him a bunch of soda, and let him watch TV, not really thinking he'd be at the station that long. That was a big mistake, because soon after, the kid went berserk. I mean, he was so hyper that he probably could have walked upside-down on the ceiling.

My partner and I got called back to the ER because we forgot to sign off on some stuff. It had to be taken care of *right then*, and there was no getting around it.

We didn't know what we were going to do with this kid, until my partner and I came up with a genius idea.

See, we put a blood pressure cuff on the kid's wrist and then tied a bunch of leads to the cuff, which created one of those leash things that parents put on their kids when they go to the zoo.

The nurses and patients kind of gave us some weird looks, but it worked.

--N.R.
Nevada

Another Day in the Neighborhood

Just because I don't work in a hospital anymore, doesn't mean I still don't witness the absurdity people have to offer…or end up being 'that' person.

Right as two police cars pulled in front of my house and parked, someone called and asked, "Isn't Mr. Smith your neighbor?"

Mr. Smith, my other neighbors, and I get together for barbeques, talk routinely, and just a few days ago, he came in my house (that he's been in several times before) to do some handyman work. He's always seemed quite nice, although he may have shown a little bit of a wild streak when he got worked up over something.

"Yeah," I said. "The cops are here. What did he do now?"

"I don't know," the person said, "but it's really bad."

I shrugged it off and continued preparing my taxes. I was too busy sobbing as I watched my money disappear, that I guess I never noticed how the two officers outside never left. Instead, more officers showed up, and more phone calls flooded in. Apparently, nobody knew if Mr. Smith was home, but everyone said the same thing: he was wanted for something *bad*. We're not talking 'bad,' as in, "Hey, Mr. Smith ran a red light in front of a school." We're talking 'bad,' as in, "You should call 911 if you see him."

"How do you know all this?" I asked.

"Well, it's on the scanner," someone said. "You should turn it on. It's crazy out there today."

Within seconds of turning on the scanner, I heard officers talking about Mr. Smith. There was a BOLO called for him several times. Officers were advised to exercise extreme caution if they located him. Officers blocked the alleyway and side streets, giving Mr. Smith only one way in or out.

I turned the scanner off and continued with my business. Obviously, Mr. Smith couldn't have been at his home, or they would have already apprehended him, right?

So, here I was, making one of those fun and not-at-all stressful (eye roll) phone calls to my student loan lender, when I saw officers continue to walk in front of my house. No big deal. They'd been doing that for hours. The business across the street was still in operation, people had still been walking their dogs, mail had been delivered, and another neighbor took out his trash. It didn't appear that anyone was in immediate danger.

"And do you have a copy of your paperwork?" the operator asked me.

I searched my desk.

"I must have left it in the car after I opened the mail," I admitted.

"It would be helpful if we could review that together. Are you able to retrieve it?"

"Oh yeah," I said, "no problem."

I pushed through the swarm of dogs and cats to get to the front door. I was only going to be a hot minute, so I didn't even slip on house shoes. I opened the door, stepped out on the porch, and mindlessly closed the door behind me.

"Get back inside," an officer ordered in a rush.

A sea of SWAT officers stood in front of my house, armed with long guns, a barricade ram, and a K9 unit.

Well, that was a no-brainer. I'd just go back inside, no problem.

It *was* a problem for me, because I live my life mixed up between clumsiness and bad luck.

I jiggled the door handle.

"You need to go inside," the officer repeated.

"Oh my God," I repeated at least ten times in five seconds, as my breathing became rapid and my heart raced.

"Are you okay?" the operator asked me.

"No!" I exclaimed. "The SWAT team is here for my neighbor, and I can't get back in my house!"

"What's the problem?" another officer asked me.

"I locked myself out," I shouted in a panic.

My brain gave a futile order to keep trying the door, and everything around me faded out.

Seconds later, I heard what sounded like an explosion. It was loud, and I gasped. My dogs were on the other side of the door, barking and growling.

"Are you okay?" the operator asked. "I'm still here. Are you okay?"

Between the dogs and the noise from next door, I could hardly hear the operator or myself.

"I don't know," I blurted out. "It's just supposed to be another weekday!"

I glanced over in panic, and a smoke-like substance surrounded the neighbor's house from a canister they had launched inside.

"I'm locked out," I said. At that point, I don't think I was talking to anyone in particular, as much as I was just repeating what I already knew.

"The back door!" I shouted. "I let the dogs out earlier, and I don't think I locked it."

I said to the operator, "You're coming with me. I need to go inside."

"I'm still here," the operator said. "I'm not hanging up."

Two of my dogs heard the gate open, and they were barking wildly at the back door. I hurried inside, and the sounds of the barks were deafening.

"Are you inside?" the operator asked.

My mind started playing reels of news footage of standoffs and shootouts. I didn't even know if Mr. Smith was home, but it's all I could imagine happening.

"I'm going to the bathroom," I said in a rush. "It's the only room that doesn't have a window facing that house."

As I was pacing the bathroom, something in my brain clicked, and I asked calmly, "Can we go over that paperwork, even though I don't have my copy?"

The operator seemed stunned and said, "Uh…yes."

There was no way I was hanging up on the nicest operator I'd ever spoken to from the lender, and the matter was pressing—obviously so pressing that I couldn't be bothered with what was happening outside.

Friends and neighbors were blowing up my phone. The call waiting beep interrupted the operator every few seconds, and I could hear my iPod dinging from all the messages coming in. I handled business with the operator and left the bathroom.

Ordinarily, I would have never gone outside if I thought police presence would lead to a SWAT invasion. I don't generally care what any of my neighbors do or don't do, as long as they leave me out of whatever is happening. In this case, I guess I kind of threw myself right in the mix.

To top it all off, I was still in my mismatched pajamas, so I essentially locked myself outside in mismatched pjs, barefoot, while there was a raid going on next door.

How's that for luck?

They Say the Darndest Things

I work in Triage, so at my hospital, patients see me before anyone else. After I assess the patient, I will either take them to a room for immediate treatment, or I will ask them to speak to a registration clerk while they are waiting to be called for treatment.

One day, a woman came in with three children. One child was probably about 10. She was walking on her own. Mom held the hand of a 2 to 3-year-old boy, and she held an infant. The infant's nose was red and snotty, but mom wasn't looking too hot, either. I honestly didn't know which to expect as my patient.

I motioned for the family to come to my work area.

"Go sit in the waiting room," the mother told her eldest child. "Sit where I can see you, and don't talk to anyone. Don't touch anything."

She handed the child her phone and said, "No videos. You can play games, but you'd better not let me find out you were on YouTube or the internet."

So far, so good.

Mom stepped in my office and sat down.

"What brings you here today?" I asked.

In the loudest shout ever, her toddler hollered, "When she yelled at me, she went 'ACHOO!' and peed her pants! And then she thought she was going to fart, but she pooped! She pooped, right in her pants!"

Visitors passing through the lobby, recently-discharged patients, our registration clerk, and a few people in the nearby waiting room laughed. One man laughed so hard that he choked on his drink and I had to leave the Triage room to make sure he wasn't choking to death.

I returned to my office and awkwardly asked the woman, "So, uh, having some stomach bug symptoms today?"

Still as red as a Camaro, she shook her head and said, "No. I got my finger stuck on the loose door frame."

She shifted the baby from one arm to the other and unwrapped a dish towel she had around her finger. Her nail was missing, and she had a deep gash in her fingertip.

I couldn't stop myself from chuckling at her son's excuse for her being in the emergency room.

She must have been in a rush to explain because she said, "It was just leakage, from giving birth. And the other part, well...I misjudged."

We went straight back, and mom received a few sutures. She, Mr. Big-Mouth, and the other kids left within a half hour.

--C.E.

Connecticut

I Have Little Arms

The funniest run of my career was when I was dispatched to an ankle injury.

When we arrived, we found a female in one of those blow-up T-Rex costumes, lying on the sidewalk, crying. Her friends surrounded her, and they were still arguing over whether or not they should remove the roller skate from her foot.

I guess they had been trying to film a funny video in hopes that it would go viral on YouTube and social media, only for the girl to trip over a stick.

She snapped her ankle and required a few screws and surgery, but it was hilarious to have to transport a dinosaur to the ER.

The best part of all of it was when they asked for identification. She kept squirming and said, "I can't reach my pocket!"

--M.K.
Pennsylvania

Back to Reality

I used to be terribly rude to everyone, and I think it was just because I felt overwhelmed with my new job.

Charge called me one day, and she asked, "Err…Hey, what's wrong with that patient you just signed in?"

"Well, if you'd take two seconds to read it, you'd know," I snapped. "Shortness of breath. How hard is that to figure out?"

"Honey, maybe you should lose the attitude and take a look at your screen," Charge said.

I looked down.

'Djpyumtff oh mytryj' is what I typed, when I misaligned my fingers to the keys.

I changed the complaint in the computer and went to talk to Charge in private. She was really nice to me and said that everyone could tell I was having a hard time with the workload and especially with abuse complaints. She said I could come talk to here whenever I needed to vent, and she said a lot of nurses offered their ears, too.

That moment really changed my outlook at work. I realized that if I was being rude to my coworkers, I was probably being rude to patients, too. I didn't want someone to come in, suffering from an illness or injury, and feel like they were inconveniencing or scaring me.

So, I put on my big girl panties and accepted that the world isn't this place filled with puppies and rainbows like I always thought it was before I started working in the hospital, and I started seeing things for what they were: tragic and unfortunate, but not worthy of a major depressive episode or being hateful to everyone.

--K.T.
New Jersey

Relocating the Fight

It was clear on of our RNs was having marital trouble, even before she vented to the other nurses. She was in a foul mood for weeks. As details emerged, we learned the RN's husband believed she was having an affair because their sex life had diminished. However, she admitted to her coworkers that she no longer felt comfortable getting naked in front of her husband, after he had too much to drink, critiqued her body, and commented on her sister's and neighbor's physique. Her husband, once sober, denied ever finding the neighbor or sister sexually attractive, but he did stand by his comments regarding his wife's body, specifically her 'gross' stomach that was 'ruined' by stretch marks, and 'saggy' breasts. This was especially painful for her because her child was stillborn a year prior. She then began showing signs of abuse, but she refused to comment on the bruises.

One day, the RN was late for her shift. Her coworkers were becoming quite worried for her wellbeing, especially after they repeatedly called her and received no answer. It was terribly busy as well, so tensions were already high. Even I was asked to stay over, and physicians at this facility are rarely asked to clock overtime.

The Head Nurse asked me what we should do, so I explained that I felt it was necessary to notify the House Supervisor of the RN's absence. The RN had never been late for work, so the fact that she was nearly an hour late was troubling. I suggested mentioning the RN's marital problems and asking for an officer to perform a welfare check.

As the nurse was making the phone call to the House Supervisor, our RN walked in, drenched from head to toe.

"I'm sorry," I remember her saying. "John threw my phone in the dishwater, so I couldn't call."

"Are you okay?" someone asked. "Do you need to take the day off?"

I think the offer was real, but everyone was hoping she didn't say no. Another RN had called in sick, and they were already having difficulty replacing her. If they were down two RNs, it would make for an even more horrible shift.

The RN laughed and waved it off. "No, no. I just need a minute to change my clothes. He took my car keys, so I had to walk."

"You walked here?" another RN exclaimed. "Don't you live, like, a few miles from here?"

"Something like that," she replied. "It's no big deal. Look, I'm sorry that I'm late. I can stay over, take extra shifts—anything. Just don't write me up, please."

The RN changed her scrubs and came back to work.

I think we saw about 25 patients in a half hour. It was busy, busy, run, run.

One of the brand-new intake clerks came to my desk and asked, "Um, do you know a Nurse Jane?"

I nodded and said, "I just sent her to discharge a patient."

"Oh," he said.

"Want me to give her a message?"

"Uh, yeah," he said, shifting nervously. "Can you tell her that her husband is in the lobby? And, uh, I think he's really mad."

I instructed the young man to go back to his desk and tell the RN's husband that she was with a patient, but we would notify her that he was waiting.

I contemplated calling security, but I thought I would give the RN that option. In no way did I wish to overstep.

I carefully viewed the monitor that streamed security footage from the lobby. I leaned in and attempted to get a good look at the RN's husband. He was holding a large cardboard box.

As I could hear him shouting from the lobby, I continued to watch the monitor. This man opened the box and started throwing sex toys at the intake clerk and around the lobby. I immediately called security.

The RN's husband told officers that he brought all his wife's toys, and also bought her more, since she was no longer interested in 'putting out.' He denied abusive behavior, but the RN confessed to officers that her husband had beaten her before her shift. She showed officers and they took pictures of the bruises that mostly covered her back.

I am happy to tell you that Jane filed for divorce from her abusive husband. She was mortified over the sex toy incident, but nobody teased her about it or gossiped behind her back; everyone felt sorry for her.

Jane and I started dating almost a few months her divorce was finalized, and I proposed to her three months later. That may not seem like a great deal of time, but we knew each other from work, which I suspect helped us hurry it along. That, and well, it just felt 'right.' We've been married for 14 years next month and have three children.

--R.L.D., M.D.
Illinois

<u>Isolation</u>

I am not a nurse, but I do work in the ER as a unit clerk. Because administration wanted staff with knowledge of medical terminology and versed in emergent situations, my coworkers and I work rotating shifts as ER registration.

One day, I was working that position, when a young woman staggered inside. She was bleeding from the mouth, was covered in burns, and I could barely see any of her natural skin pigment because she was bruised from head to toe. Chunks of her hair were torn out and also burned off. To this day, I have no idea how she made it to the hospital or how she walked inside, but as soon as she passed through the revolving door, she collapsed.

I first called to the treatment area, to the unit clerk's phone. It rang four times before the call 'ricocheted' to the next available line, which belonged to our physician, a fresh-out-of-school, doe-eyed, naïve, know-it-all with a bad attitude.

He picked up the phone and I could hear him complaining to someone that he was tired of the 'help's' calls ringing to his phone. I knew he had a habit of placing calls on hold without notifying the caller, so I had to think fast.

I screamed forcefully, "Don't you dare put me on hold. Send help to the front NOW."

I wish I could say that this man obeyed my order after he abruptly hung up on me, but he didn't. I gave it about thirty seconds, but when help didn't arrive, I bolted to the back, stood in the corridor, and shouted, "I need everyone available right now!"

Three RNs and one pediatrician (on his way back to his floor after an ER consult) hurried to the front with a stretcher.

As I stood by and watched the four carefully lift the patient, I could smell her burned flesh and hair. I could also smell gasoline and another substance. Unfortunately, this meant she had to be rushed to the decon shower before being admitted to the treatment area.

I was ordered to call a code, arrange a flight transfer, and call law enforcement. As I was doing this, I could hear the woman shrieking from the decon area. The shrieking continued down the hall, as the patient was transferred to a room.

Minutes later, one of my friends came inside. He was calm and collected, as usual.

"Hey," he greeted me with a smile.

"Hi, John," I said. "What are you doing here?"

He pointed to the treatment area doors and said, "I just came to see if you have someone back there right now."

"I can look up a name for you," I answered.

"Jane Smith is who I'm looking for," he said.

I checked the ER admission log on my computer screen. Jane Smith was the patient who'd just come in, and she was listed as a private patient, meaning I could not verify that she was there.

"Sorry," I said. "I don't have anyone by that name."

He leaned in and asked, "Are you sure? I just watched her come in. I just need to talk to her."

I felt that I needed to ask more questions, but I couldn't. When a patient is listed as private, I can give no indication of his/her presence, no matter what. I didn't know why I felt it at the time, but I felt like John was trying to trick me into confirming Jane's admission, and I felt as if he was pressuring me.

I shrugged. "Sorry, John. I don't have a patient listed by that name."

He took a deep breath and then grinned. "Okay, okay," he said. "Hey, are we still on for that cookout this weekend?"

I nodded.

"And I've been meaning to ask you, did you watch *Game of Thrones* the other night?"

The phone rang, and I said as I pointed, "Sorry, John. I really can't talk right now."

"No problem, no problem," he said.

I felt uneasy, but I didn't know why. John and I had been friends for maybe four or five years. I met him through my neighbors, who knew him from work. He was really an outstanding guy. He volunteered at the Humane Society and rang the donation bell for The Salvation Army at Christmastime. He was a single guy with no kids. He'd dated around, but he just hadn't found 'the one.' He had a steady job that paid well, he owned a nice home in a nice neighborhood, and he was friendly to everyone. My neighbors and I went over to John's for cookouts almost every weekend during the summers. He visited our homes frequently. I have never admitted this before because I am still embarrassed and ashamed, but John and I had a bit of a romantic relationship. It was more of a hookup that occurred a week prior to this. The only reason it didn't continue is that I had just left a relationship, and I wasn't ready. John was great. He was sweet, caring, charming…He was everything you'd want a man to be. It just wasn't the right time to be getting in another relationship. He understood and said we could be friends, that if I changed my mind, he'd be there.

I was still engaged with the caller when I saw three police cars enter the parking lot.

John glanced to the lot and then lightly tapped the counter.

"I'll see you around, Sweetheart," he said to me.

He pulled his ballcap securely around his head and walked out. He even greeted the officers on his way out.

The second unit clerk raced to the front, out of breath, moments after I allowed the officers to the back. John got in his vehicle and drove away.

"That man you were talking to!" the unit clerk gasped. "That was John, right?"

I nodded and blushed a little. She knew he was my friend because she had attended one of our cookouts. She'd been pressuring me to date him for the longest time. I thought she had seen him on the security footage and wanted to gossip.

"The lady is saying that he did this to her," my coworker continued. "They're getting the details of the story, and then they're going after him."

What? No way. I didn't believe what my coworker just said to me. Honestly, I didn't believe her. I thought the patient was confused and gave the wrong name.

"John's not that kind of person," I said.

"Honey, the patient said it happened in his house. She gave details. According to her, he did this. He invited her over for lunch, and then he attacked her."

I still didn't believe it. There was just no way sweet John could do something like that. No way.

An officer returned to the lobby and told me the patient was a no-go. The only people allowed in her room were her nurses, doctors, and officers. No non-essential staff could go in. No visitors. I was told I could not go in. We were supposed to confirm information with information collected by officers, and then leave her file alone. Officers weren't worried about insurance or anything like that, because here we have an abuse fund that covers bills for victims. I've been working here a long time, and this is the only time a patient has been restricted.

The officer then asked to use my desk phone, and he called someone. Dispatch put out an all-officers BOLO for John and said he should be considered armed and dangerous.

As the shift dragged on, details leaked from staff and officers. John invited the patient over. She knew him from work and was thrilled that he wanted to cook her lunch. She said they'd been talking and sexting for a month (which overlapped with the time I had been intimate with him, which left me even more shocked and angry), and that entire time, he'd been trying to get her to come over. John took her to the basement, beat her with a metal pipe, sexually abused her, and then poured gasoline and paint thinner on her, before setting her on fire. The list of her injuries is too long and gruesome to cite, but she was missing most of her teeth and had several internal injuries that required surgery, not to mention her external injuries, which required a burn unit. If the patient did not die, she was looking at several months of rehabilitation. John placed the woman in the back seat of his vehicle and planned to dump her in the conservation area to die. She ran when he stopped at a corner market to buy cleaner to clean evidence out of his vehicle.

I threw up when I heard all the details emerge. My mind was racing, and all I could think was, 'Why her and not me?' I was living in a prison as thoughts of being intimate with him played over and over in my head. I experienced the full spectrum of emotions.

John was apprehended two hours later, after he took officers on a high-speed chase and attempted to take a hostage.

When I got home that evening, my neighbors were waiting on my porch.

"Did you hear about John?" they asked. "We heard he got arrested."

I kind of shrugged.

"We saw his charges."

"I heard they were pretty bad," I choked.

"Yeah," the husband said, "I think he could be looking at hard time. What a shame. He doesn't deserve it."

"He doesn't deserve it?" I blurted out.

The wife agreed and said, "Whatever he did, I'm sure the person was asking for it."

I played dumb and said, "Well, I don't know about that. I don't know what happened, but the charges you just listed are pretty serious."

"Well, we'll hear his side when he gets out," the husband said.

"Yeah," said the wife, "I'm already thinking that we should have a party for when he's released."

I thought I was going to pass out on my porch as I listened to these two talk.

"I don't think he's getting out for a long time, and I don't think he should, either," I said.

"Oh, don't be that way," the wife said to me. "You can't hate someone, based on what others said they did. I mean, if I went ballistic and hit someone in the park, would you still be scared of me?"

I hesitated.

She continued, "John's never done anything to you or me. I have no reason to be afraid of him. He's still my friend."

"We just don't know all the details," I said.

"No," said the husband, "but you're already judging him. He slipped up and hit a woman, so what?"

I wanted to scream that John didn't just slap this patient and realize that he'd hit a woman. He beat her, sexually assaulted her, doused her in gasoline, lit her on fire, *and* attempted to dump her to die.

But, I couldn't say those things.

Over the next few days, my neighbors and friends were still rooting for John. His bond had been set at half-a-million-dollars, cash only.

When a group of my neighbors and friends approached me and asked me to donate to a collection they were raising to bail him out of jail, I politely declined.

As soon as I declined, I became the odd one out. Everyone on my street stopped talking to me. Friends I'd met at our cookouts, they wouldn't talk to me if we saw each other in the grocery store. As far as they were concerned, I was just the heartless bitch who wouldn't give John a chance.

Nobody really thinks about these things when they meet a healthcare employee. I never did. But, when you know a nurse or a doctor, a tech or a secretary, you don't know what secrets they're hiding. You don't know that they knew Mr. Smith from three houses down came in for an STD check because he was cheating on his wife. You don't know that they knew Mrs. Smith was diagnosed with cancer at three in the morning, when she came in for dizziness. But we know those things, and we have to walk around with secrets stirring inside us.

Don't get me wrong, I don't care that I have to know these secrets and protect them. That's not the point. My point is that sometimes our secrets could make a difference in how people are viewed. You would think that John's charges and bond would have been enough for the neighbors and my friends to have realized that John wasn't the man we thought he was. If they knew the details, I thought, surely, they would change their minds, instead of already planning to bring him in their homes, instead of living in a make-believe world where John was set free.

More than a year has passed. John was sentenced to many decades in prison. He won't have a shot at parole until he's in his 80s. My neighbors never talked to me again, and neither did half my friends. Some came around and realized that John must have done something terrible to receive such a sentence. Others were still in denial. For example, I would be in the backyard gardening, when my neighbors would loudly talk to one another and claim John was a victim of police evidence-planting, or that charges were brought against him falsely. I learned to ignore my neighbors when they talked like that.

I basically had to start from scratch when it came to friends outside of work. I started talking to some coworkers and they said they'd experienced similar situations in the past, but never so severe. They said to ignore what people had to say, because I knew the truth about what John had done.

This job can leave you feeling isolated, I've learned that. You'll learn things about people that nobody else knows, and even when it comes down to a need to use those details to explain why you can't support someone, you can't. Details of the patient's abuse were never made public, and even if they were, I couldn't talk about anything I'd seen because it is my job to uphold patient privacy. I basically have to accept that I will lose friends, or I have to pretend that I agree with them. I can't do that. I can't pretend to support someone, knowing they committed such a heinous crime.

On a positive note, I made more medical friends, so we've bonded and understand each other better than I could have ever dreamed of relating with my neighbors and non-medical friends. The patient, by the way, lived. She was afraid John would be released from jail, so she changed her name and moved.

--Initials and location withheld at request

Eek!

I was dispatched to a residence, after a driver called 911 to report that someone on drugs was in a backyard, screaming, and flailing about at 02:30.

I was just down the block, so I reached the residence in under a minute, just as a female was approaching the home's front door.

I exited my vehicle and stopped the female.

"Is everything okay here?" I asked.

I saw that she had something in her right hand, and I started thinking that maybe this was not her residence. I ordered her to drop what she was holding, as I reached for my flashlight and my other hand hovered over my weapon.

She dropped what she had in her hand, and when I shined the light on her, she had tears streaming down her cheeks.

"My night just keeps getting better and better," she mumbled.

"We received a call that someone was just in the backyard, behaving erratically. Were you out here screaming and waving your arms?"

She nodded.

"Have you been drinking tonight?" I asked. "Have you been taking drugs?"

"No!" she exclaimed.

"Are you injured?" I asked.

She shook her head.

I pointed my flashlight to the ground and saw a transparent igloo-looking thing.

"I caught a mouse," she said, nodding toward the apparatus on the ground. "When I brought it out and released it, the thing ran up my leg and then up my shirt."

"That's what you were screaming about?" I asked.

"Yes!" she shouted, now sobbing. "It was in my bra. I was trying to get it out. Am I going to jail?"

"Not tonight," I said with a chuckle.

I told her to have a good night, and I turned to go back to my car.

"Wait," she said.

I turned around.

This woman looked so afraid as she said, "I have two more traps inside. Can you help me release the mice? I hate mice. I just don't think I can handle trying to let more go tonight."

I went inside, grabbed two more traps from the woman's laundry room, and I released the mice in the alley behind the house.

"Try to get some sleep," I told her.

"And, hey," I said, "you might want to get a cat."

--C.W.
Indiana

<u>Stereotypes</u>

We were dispatched to a residence for a complaint of an incident with a pit bull, and I didn't know what to expect, really. I have never owned a pit, but a lot of my friends have them. Some of my friends' dogs are downright crazy and mean, but the other dogs are nice and cuddly. We'd responded to a lot of pit attacks in the past, so I think I imagined that we were going to arrive on scene and witness a mauled victim and a snarling dog pulling at its chain to get loose and kill. Dispatch told us a child called 911 to report that his mother needed help, mentioned the dog, was able to said 'pit bull,' and then hung up.

When we arrived, a child around the age of three met us at the door.

"Is your mommy hurt?" I asked.

The child nodded. He looked like he'd been crying.

"Can you take us to your mommy?"

The boy nodded again and took my partner's hand. As he guided us through the house and upstairs, we were on high alert for a dog.

We went upstairs and were escorted through the master bedroom and to the master bathroom, where we found a pregnant female lying on the floor. She was sobbing in the dark.

My partner stayed in the bedroom with the child, while I knelt beside the patient.

"Were you attacked?" I asked.

"Huh?" the patient mumbled.

"Your son called 911 and said you needed help because of your dog. Were you attacked?"

"No," the woman said.

She groaned and sat up just enough to vomit.

According to the patient, her pit bull was passing gas, and since she was pregnant, the smell made her sick. She stuck the dog in the back yard and then spent the next 30 minutes vomiting, which brought on a migraine. Her son became scared and called 911.

The patient did request medical transport. Her neighbor came over to check on her as we loaded her in the ambulance, and she asked the neighbor to watch her son and call her husband.

I tell ya, I felt like the weight of expectation and fear was lifted from my shoulders. I'm glad the run didn't involve a mauling, even though I guess it technically involved a pit bull gas attack.

--G.K.

Kentucky

Play Ball!

My partner and I had to respond to a patient experiencing chest pain. Our patient lived in a busy apartment complex, on the third floor.

When we pulled in the parking lot, we couldn't park in a traditional manner, as most cars park between painted lines. The spots were too compact for our large vehicle, and even if we did park there, we wouldn't have been able to reverse without hitting the row of cars behind us. Unfortunately, our only option was to park between a row of cars, which essentially blocked in both rows. We know this would be an inconvenience for residents, but we did not anticipate being on scene for more than a few minutes, especially since the building had an elevator and the patient had a heart history. (For us, this means the patient knew something was wrong, so it would be an in and out run for us.)

We loaded our patient to a stretcher and made it back to the parking lot in just a few minutes. If I had to guess, I would say we were out of our ambulance for roughly six to eight minutes, if that.

As we were approaching the ambulance, my partner and I immediately noticed a sports car that was parked so closely to our vehicle that we would be unable to open the doors to load our patient.

This, of course, pissed us off, but we didn't see anyone in the driver's seat, so we didn't know who we'd confront.

The driver's seat was empty because the male driver, maybe 22-years-old, was on the driver's side of the ambulance, hitting it with a metal baseball bat. He was also screaming threats and obscenities.

My partner tried to reason with the guy, but the guy turned his attention from the ambulance to my partner. He chased my partner with the bat until my partner backed off. Then, the man continued wailing on the side of our vehicle. In a span of seconds, the man knocked off our side mirror and busted the headlights on the driver's side.

He wasn't blocked in, but he was blocked *out.* He was furious because our vehicle was blocking his designated parking spot, and he thought we were acting 'entitled' by blocking the reserved spot that cost him $25 a month.

I was on my cell phone with dispatch, when the man got a little too carried away with beating up the ambulance.

He drew back and took a deep breath before he swung at our vehicle for the umpteenth time.

This is when it got *really* interesting.

The bat hit the side of our ambulance and bounced off. It looked as if the man was trying to control the bounce by drawing back to take another back-to-back swing, but the bat had other plans. It whipped around and hit the patient in the back of the head. His eyes rolled back, and he fell to the ground, unconscious.

"Oh my," said our heart patient.

I was laughing so hard that I couldn't even tell dispatch what happened. My partner took my cell phone and tried to explain the situation, but he couldn't stop laughing either.

Finally, our heart patient snatched the phone out of my partner's hand and told dispatch, "Kiddo knocked himself out cold with a ball bat. Think you can get someone out here soon, so that I don't die in a parking lot?"

Not only did a backup medic crew arrive, but the cops also showed up. The man's vehicle was towed at his expense, and he was placed under arrest after he was medically cleared.

Luckily, our patient's chest pain was determined to be non-life-threatening, and he never took his frustration out on us.

--L.C.
Florida

Dive In

To boost morale, we sometimes rent out the pool at our park and hold department/family parties in there. Our department (Pediatrics) usually performs better following a party, and they're fun to bring my kids to, so I've never minded them.

I wasn't feeling very well prior to one party, but I thought getting in the water and floating around while my kids were off playing would help me feel better.

Not thinking, I jumped in the water with my cover-up on. I crocheted it from cotton and used double strands in some places, so it was kind of heavy and uncomfortable in the water.

I got out of the pool, took my cover up off, and got back in the water.

Everyone was staring at me.

I looked down and realized I had accidentally pulled my bandeau top off when I pulled off my cover up.

There I was, topless, while all my coworkers, their kids and spouses, and even our HR manager looked at me like I was crazy.

I hurried out of the pool and scrambled to put my top back on. As soon as I did, a little girl patted my leg, looked up at me, and said, "Don't worry. My mommy's boobies are floppy, too."

The child's mother, a night shift nurse, choked on her drink and rushed over from her table to grab her daughter.

We left soon after that. My kids were at that age where everything I did was embarrassing, so they cried the whole way home, saying I 'ruined their lives.'

I couldn't look my coworkers in the eye for weeks.

--M.A.
Florida

The weirdest call I was ever dispatched to was a complaint of 'nipple bitten off by bird.'

Seriously, I guess this lady was naked and feeding her parrot, when it went nuts and yanked her nipple off.

Her husband called 911 and was standing in the driveway with her nipple in a Ziploc bag when we pulled up.

That was an insane shift.

--H.A.

Nevada

<u>Do As I Say, Not As I Do</u>

A few readers want to share some advice with the world. I feel like I'm doing a public service by passing the word to others.

Should you ever stumble home after a long night of tequila shots and purple hooter shooters and get the bright idea to karate-chop your 2"-thick wooden cutting board in half, don't.

I puked out of a combination of being plastered and in pain, hit my head on the stove, and I fractured the hell out of my hand.

My roommate was drunk, too, so we had to call his mom at four in the morning to drive us to the hospital. She lectured us the whole way there and back. The hospital gave me a neon orange cast, which I likened to a scarlet letter, because everyone seemed to take one look at me and know I got it by doing something stupid. I was also in nursing school at that time and barely graduated because of complications with my hand.

The cutting board, by the way, was fine. It seemed to play the 'I'm rubber and you're glue game' and reflect any damage I was doing to it back on me.

--N.E.

Massachusetts

If you are at work and are too embarrassed to call out to your all-male office for toilet paper because you don't want them to know that you, the only female employee, were pooping, don't use bleach wet wipes as an alternative to toilet paper, especially after you've shaved all your private areas.

I stood up and screamed so loud when my bikini area and butthole started burning that one of the guys thought I was in trouble. When I didn't respond to his knocks on the door, he kicked the door down, which hit me in the back and pushed me down into the toilet. My face landed in the toilet bowl and when I tried to grab something, I flushed the toilet, effectively giving myself a 'swirly.'

It wasn't until I was trying to pull up my underwear and pants that I realized I had cut my other hand on something when all the commotion went down.

I had to go to the ER for nine stitches.

I wish my coworker would've lied for me and said that I saw a snake or something, but he wouldn't. This story is his favorite to tell around the office, and he finds a way to bring it up in almost any conversation.

--A.J.
Tennessee

My wife and I were attending an open house on a property we'd eyed from roadside. You would think that a couple trying to sell their home would be cheerful and polite, but these people were assholes, plain and simple. They made a bunch of snide, backhanded comments that suggested that my wife and I were not good enough for the neighborhood, couldn't afford the property, and that list goes on and on.

My last straw was when we were going to the backyard. I held the patio storm door open for the seller's wife, but she apparently thought she was above saying a simple 'thank you' to me, and instead, she gave me a condescending glance that seemed to size me up as her door attendant. Completely fed up, I let the door go. Hold your own damn door, Your Highness.

Well, a storm was rolling in, and the wind grabbed the door from her side. It slammed right into my face, and I was bleeding everywhere.

My wife, a neurosurgeon, took a quick look at me and said it looked like my nose was broken. I was also missing one of my front teeth.

ER trip. Dental appointment. Nothing compared to the instant reprimand from the universe telling me to be nice, even when others aren't.

We did *not* purchase that house. I mean, we were still thinking about it, but then we heard sewage backed up into all the home's sinks and showers, due to a collapsed line that would cost about $9,000 (on the low-end) to fix.

Guess they got what was coming to them, too.

--D.R.
Maine

If you're ever in the mood to paint your nails, but you're too drunk to sit up properly, just wait till later.

I somehow managed to drop bright blue polish in my eye. I remember that it hurt, but I was so drunk that I kind of wiped some of it away and then blacked out.

I had to visit an optometrist, who basically called me stupid as he used some kind of drops and tool to kind of scrape the polish off.

The damage was done, though, and the polish scratched and damaged my cornea so badly that I can hardly see out of my left eye.

That, by far, was the most idiotic thing I have ever done while intoxicated, and it pretty much ruined my life.

--N.S.
Mississippi

It *is* possible to check how hot the iron is before putting it away by hovering your hand over it, rather than just pressing your palm to the metal.

I learned that the hard way.

Second-degree burns and a doctor actually asking, "Are you stupid?"

--N.H.
Missouri

There is a reason items have warning labels. If something tells you it's not for internal use or consumption, pay attention to that warning.

My patient came in with chemical burns to her vaginal cavity because she tried to douche with the oil in one of those air freshener plug-ins.

When I asked her why she did this, she said she really liked the Hawaiian scent, and she thought she could impress her partner if her vagina smelled like a mixture of coconut and pineapple.

She was treated and advised not to have sex for 4-6 weeks.

--T.K.
Arizona

Don't stick stuff in your penis.

As a male nurse, I cringe when my patients present with pen caps, straws, syringes, thermometers, Q-tips, and even caulk stuck in their weenies.

I have noticed most of these patients present between 03:00-06:00, so my advice would be this: If you have an urge to stick something up your wee, sleep it off.

--M.M.

Think ahead if you're on your period.

I suffer from heavy cycles and usually have to use extra-thick pads or double up. I didn't remember to stock my locker, and I thought I could manage for the rest of my shift, so I used a pad and then wrapped a half of roll of toilet paper around the inside/outside of my panties.

My patient's kid thought it would be funny to 'de-pants' me, and everyone in the room (including the doctor) saw my makeshift pad setup.

The patient's dad told mom about it when she came back from the cafeteria, and she whooped the boy's butt. She felt so bad about it that she tried to give me a gift card to the hospital's gift shop, but I declined.

I've never forgotten to stock up on feminine products since then.

--A.W.

California

Do you know why I.T. professionals ask you if the device is plugged in and turned on when you call the help line? It's because you should make sure you're not stupid before you call and complicate things.

I was so mad that my computer wasn't working, that I lost my temper and kicked the tower that was on the floor under my desk. I don't even know how it happened, but I fractured my foot and had to wear a cast and use a scooter for months.

My computer wouldn't work because the power strip was turned off.

I was written up for unprofessional behavior, which I guess was better than getting fired.

--L.X.
Oregon

If you engage in unprotected intercourse and do not wish to become pregnant, it's better to purchase Plan B or consult your physician, rather than attempt to 'clean yourself out' with bleach, followed by a chaser of ammonia.

Our patient sustained severe chemical burns and was transferred out.

The patient's boyfriend called 911, after the patient passed out from the gas the chemicals created during their interaction.

I wish I made this up.

--T.U.
South Carolina

If you wear long johns under your scrubs, make sure you remember to put scrubs on.

I didn't realize I was only wearing long john bottoms until I was half-way to the front door of the ED. I had to call my boss from the parking lot and ask her to run me out a pair of loaner scrubs because I didn't have time to go back home, and I knew I didn't have my backup pair in my locker.

I went back to my car and waited for her to bring the pants out. I lied and said I had spilled coffee all over myself and that I was too embarrassed to walk inside.

I guess that's what I get for getting dressed at 04:00.

--H.N.
Indiana

Boogie Nights

When I was in nursing school (age 25), a bunch of us got together and went to this sleazy bar that had a stripper pole up on a stage. My classmates brought along some guys, and I thought I would impress a guy I thought was cute if I got up on stage and started showing how sexy I could be. I'm blaming this idea on the ridiculous amount of alcohol I'd consumed.

I got up on stage and thought I was doing okay. The music was loud, and everyone was cheering me on.

Everything was great…well, right up to the point that I tried to hang upside down on the pole.

I fell off the pole, hit my head on the stage, and then fell off the stage.

I broke both my arms, had to take an ambulance to the hospital, and I had to drop out of nursing school for that semester, which almost got me kicked out of the program.

And the guy I was trying to impress? He was still in high school! He got in the bar by using a fake ID.

--O.G.

Michigan

I was speed-walking through the ER before my shift on Rehab started, just like I do every morning, when I slipped on something slick.

It was human poop.

I slipped on human poop and had to use crutches for four months.

With luck this bad, rest assured that I will certainly never win the lottery.

K.E.

Kansas

Fashionistas

We received a cardiac patient from EMS, after the tourist showed symptoms of a heart attack while exploring downtown with his family.

I was at the registration desk when this elderly lady and her husband approached me. They showed me a picture of our patient, and his name was written at the bottom of the picture. It was clear the couple did not speak English.

What was hilarious about this couple was that they were both wearing shirts you would expect to see college frat boys wearing.

The woman, so old that she could barely take more than three steps at a time before needing to lean against her walker and rest, had a shirt on that read: I'm a virgin. (This shirt is old.)

Her husband's shirt was red and had a white medical cross on it. His shirt read:

Orgasm Donor, Saving Lives One F*** at a Time.

They seemed confused by my behavior because I couldn't stop laughing.

I called switchboard, and the operator paged an Oncology nurse who speaks Japanese. She escorted the family to our patient. I later asked her if she thought the couple knew what their shirts said, and she said they probably did not know. I guess their culture has a fad going on, where people like to buy shirts with English phrases on them, just because they look cool or something.

I can only imagine the looks they received while they were exploring the city!

--E.P.
Nevada

A Message from the Author

Thanks for sticking around for another book! I hope you all enjoyed the 2 for 1.

I wanted to address a few concerns readers brought up in reviews and messages. I may eventually discuss this on my social media accounts.

Firstly, I have received a miniscule amount of negative feedback for the titles of these books. Some readers have been disappointed to purchase a book and find the stories do not revolve around the title. This, obviously, excludes themed releases, such as the holiday or LEO books.

As most of you are aware by now, I take the titles from submissions. If something stands out and makes for a good title, that's what it becomes. Unfortunately, I think it would take 12 years to find every story about full moons or exercising to fill a book of stories based on the title. That many stories about one topic may read a bit stale for most readers' preference, as well.

Secondly, a few readers have mentioned similarities to some stories or have commented that the books are repetitious. I will agree. Even as I dig through submissions, I am reminded of stories from the past—even ones that never made it to the books. That's a part of being in the medical field, folks. Crazy things are not limited to San Francisco or Norfolk or Tallahassee. Some of the submissions bear similarities, but each reader possesses the knowledge and emotion that comes from his or her personal encounter with the patient in question. I guess you can say the same thing about other books and movies. For example, there are tons of zombie movies out there. Many share the same plot, but it's in the details and the presentation that makes one stand out more than the other. I never want readers to feel that they cannot share experiences because, 'Oh well, it's probably happened to a million people before me.' That may be true, but it's never happened to you. That makes an ordinary situation unique to the reader.

Other than touching down on those two points, I can't think of anything to add on a 'business level.'

I went rather slow with this edition. When you go, go, go all the time, doing what you love becomes a burden, and I never want to feel that way about writing. I actually broke my finger in the early stages of this book (which seems to have been a recurring thing in the submissions, too), so that slowed me down for a while…until I learned to type just as fast without using that finger. My thoughts right now are in Jeff Goldblum's voice from Jurassic Park, as I think, 'Writing, uh, finds a way.'

I will do my very best to keep everyone updated on future works. A faithful reader who's been around since book one suggested I post a few stories on Facebook every month, and that's an idea I'll consider. It is a smart idea!

Thank you all for your continued support. Have a great day!

Check me out on Twitter!

https://twitter.com/AuthorKerryHamm

You can also find me on Facebook, by searching for 'Author Kerry Hamm.'

Made in the USA
Las Vegas, NV
07 January 2021

15389772R00252